MOTOR

ASSESSMENT *of*

the DEVELOPING

INFANT

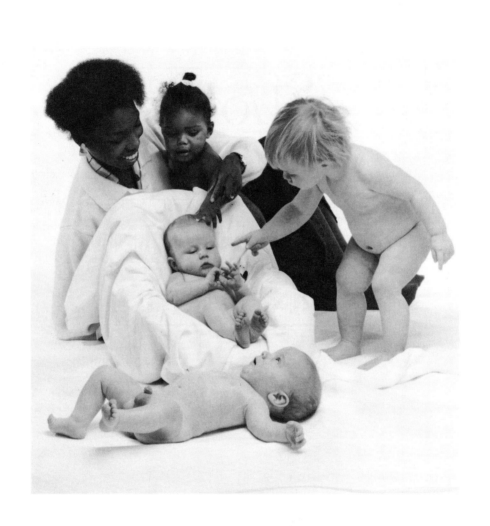

MOTOR

ASSESSMENT *of*

the DEVELOPING

INFANT

Martha C. Piper, Ph.D.
Vice-President (Research)
University of Alberta
Edmonton, Alberta
Canada

Johanna Darrah, M.Sc., P.T.
Joint Appointment
Faculty of Rehabilitation Medicine
University of Alberta
and Glenrose Rehabilitation Hospital
Edmonton, Alberta
Canada

Neil Boyce, *Photographer*

SAUNDERS
An Imprint of Elsevier

SAUNDERS

An Imprint of Elsevier

The Curtis Center
Independence Square West
Philadelphia, Pennsylvania 19106

Library of Congress Cataloging-in-Publication Data

Piper, Martha C.

Motor assessment of the developing infant / Martha C. Piper,
Johanna Darrah.

p.   cm.

ISBN-13: 978-0-7216-4307-6   ISBN-10: 0-7216-4307-8

1. Infants—Development.   I. Darrah, Johanna.
   II. Title.   [DNLM: 1. Motor Skills—in infancy & childhood.
   2. Child Development.   WE 103 P665m 1994]

RJ134.P57 1993   155.42′223—dc20

DNLM/DLC   93–24914

Motor Assessment of the Developing Infant

Permissions may be sought directly from Elsevier's Health Sciences
Rights Department in Philadelphia, PA, USA: phone: (+1) 215 239 3804,
fax: (+1) 215 239 3805, e-mail: healthpermissions@elsevier.com. You
may also complete your request on-line via the Elsevier homepage
(http://www.elsevier.com), by selecting 'Customer Support' and then
'Obtaining Permissions'.

Printed in the United States of America.

ISBN-13: 978-0-7216-4307-6
ISBN-10: 0-7216-4307-8

Last digit is the print number: 25 24 23 22 21

Contributors

· ·

Thomas O. Maguire, Ph.D.
Professor, Educational Psychology, University of Alberta, Edmonton, Alberta, Canada

Lynn Redfern, Ph.D.
Clinical Nurse Researcher, Royal Alexandra Hospital, Edmonton, Alberta, Canada

Preface

· ·

The human child is the greatest miracle of creation. Every single child, moreover, is a world of subtle secrets, a personality, a unique occurrence, never to be repeated on this earth.

Alva Myrdal, as quoted by Sissela Bok in *Alva Myrdal, A Daughter's Memoir,*
Radcliffe Biography Series, 1991 (p. 129)

As Sissela Bok highlights in her biography of her extraordinary mother, Nobel Prize winner Alva Myrdal, the relationships between parents and children are constantly changing. Roles, expectations, and needs continue to evolve, changing with age and time. Infants become children; children become adults; adults become parents; parents become children. Nothing is certain, nothing is static, nothing is predictable. Such is the case of child development in general and infant motor development in particular.

The splendor of infancy is perhaps best expressed and celebrated by observing the infant explore and discover the world through the development of movement. The demonstrable skill of movement provides tangible evidence that the infant is evolving, becoming a personality, a unique occurrence. As with the infant's personality, the ability to move against gravity and assume an upright position evolves and matures. While movement unfolds, to a large extent in a predictable fashion, the subtleties each child brings to the process ensure that no two infants are exactly alike in how they move or evolve.

To witness the unfolding of motor skills during an infant's first two years of life contributes to the sense of wonder surrounding infant development. During these months, the motor abilities of an infant explode, so much that often it is difficult to absorb all the changes that occur. The rate of change in early motor development presents a special challenge to health care professionals involved in the assessment of infants' motor skills. Any assessment of motor skills in infancy is limited by the fact that we are forced to make a static evaluation of a dynamic process. The evolution of motor skills is a fluid, changing phenomenon, displaying many different facets that are dependent on the interaction of a myriad of variables. Factors as diverse as the motivation of the infant, the environment, the time of day, and the presence of a stranger may influence how an infant moves. When viewed from this perspective, any one evaluation of motor abilities is only an estimation of an infant's skills.

By observing the movements of over 2900 infants, all unique occurrences, we are convinced more than ever that what we do not know about infant movement far exceeds what we do know. Many aspects of motor development continue to elude us: is motor development linear or continuous, or are there ebbs and flows in the normal unfolding of motor competency? Do early motor delays portend future motor deficits, or can an infant spontaneously "catch up"? Why do some infants choose not to creep on their hands and knees? What are the prerequisites for early walking?

Despite these unanswered questions, we are convinced that "knowing" about movement in infancy is far less important than "observing" movement in infancy. The infants have continued to surprise us with their "subtle secrets" and their ability to teach us about movement, rather than the other way around.

We are grateful to our teachers. As students, we find once again that our roles are reversed. The infants are instructing us, becoming parent-like in their abilities to inform us about the secrets of movement. We have become the children, in awe of our teachers, learning from their movements, their adaptations, and their creativeness.

And so we thank all of the infants who have contributed to this undertaking and who have so graciously shared their experiences with us. More than anything they have taught us to take the cues from them, to permit them to exhibit their unique strengths and abilities, and to celebrate their ability to discover and execute the movements required by their environments.

Martha C. Piper, Ph.D.

Johanna Darrah, M.Sc., P.T.

Acknowledgments

· ·

The development of the Alberta Infant Motor Scale (AIMS) reflects the support and contribution of many individuals and organizations.

We are grateful for the financial support provided by the National Health Research and Development Program (NHRDP), Ottawa, Canada; the Children's Health Foundation of Northern Alberta, Edmonton, Alberta; and the Hospital for Sick Children Foundation, Toronto, Ontario. Without the sponsorship of these organizations, the Alberta Infant Motor Scale would never have been developed.

Drs. Lynn Redfern and Tom Maguire provided valuable support and assistance in the development of the psychometric properties of the AIMS.

We thank Drs. Tom Paton and Joe Watt for their assistance in accessing infants for assessment in the Edmonton area.

Dr. Paul Byrne was always available to evaluate critically all phases of the project and to provide support and encouragement to the team.

Cathy McLaggan drew the original drawings of the items, and although her drawings do not appear in this book, we acknowledge her talent and her patience while we struggled to get each drawing "just right."

Ed Rodgers provided his computer expertise throughout the development of the AIMS and the preparation of this book.

Many clinicians shared their knowledge of infant motor development with us. Therapists who participated in the initial generation and selection of items on the AIMS include Barbara Ashton, Faith Harckham, Elaine McInnes, Aline McMillan, Helen Riewe, and Lynda Schmidt at the Glenrose Rehabilitation Hospital, Edmonton, Alberta; and Penny Bourne, Mei Fong, Ann Gallagher, Ruth Goodchild, Nan Hawes-Bernbaum, Mary McNeil, Marg Nelson, Diane Ramalho, and Lorna Ruttan at the Calgary Children's Hospital, Calgary, Alberta. Members of the Pediatric Division of the Canadian Physiotherapy Association participated in a mail survey of the items; their input guided us in the selection and sequence of the items.

A panel of experts in pediatric physical and occupational therapy, Lois Bly, Suzann Campbell, Lyn Chandler, Linda Fetters, Sara Forsyth, and Susan Hardy, critiqued the initial items and provided valuable suggestions for yet another revision of the AIMS.

Therapists involved in the assessments of infants were Pam Acheson, Doreen Bartlett, Jean Fan, Faith Harckham, Jean McIlrath, Diana Nothof, Helen Riewe, Lynda Schmidt, and Hilary Sproule. Some of these women travelled many miles in variable weather conditions to evaluate infants throughout Alberta and we are especially grateful for their enthusiasm and fortitude.

The collection of data for the norming of the AIMS was a major collaborative task of many individuals and departments. Alberta Health, particularly the Division of Vital Statistics, was an integral part of the project, identifying infants throughout Alberta who were eligible for participation in the project. The nurses and auxiliary staff in the following health units assisted in both the recruitment of infants and the organization of the therapists' visits: Athabasca, Minburn-Vermilion, Big Country, Southeastern, Alberta West Central, Barons-Eureka-Warner, Edmonton, Red Deer, Jasper, and North Eastern. Our appointment secretary, Merle Martin, spent many hours on the telephone scheduling appointment times for the infants.

Annette Kujda, Project Co-ordinator, has kept all of us on track over the last five years. Without her suggestions, organizational skills, and commitment to the development of the AIMS, we could not have completed the project or this book.

Finally, we wish to thank all the infants and their parents who participated in the AIMS project. Over 2,900 infants were assessed during the development and norming of the AIMS; we extend our appreciation to their families for keeping their appointments and allowing therapists to observe their infants' motor development. In addition, we thank the parents of the infants who were photographed for the book. All of them were a delight, and we are fortunate to have had the opportunity to glimpse momentarily the motor development of so many infants.

Martha C. Piper, Ph.D.

Johanna Darrah, M.Sc., P.T.

Contents

ten

eleven

appendices

THEORIES OF MOTOR DEVELOPMENT

When an infant is born and thrust from the safe, homeostatic environment in utero into unfamiliar surroundings, he or she is completely dependent on others for all needs. Instantly, the infant's motor abilities change; the free movements experienced in utero are restricted by gravity. Instead of stepping, somersaulting, and rolling, the neonate cannot even control the position of the head. Over the next 12 months, a motor metamorphosis occurs, and the infant masters all the motor skills necessary for independence in this new environment.

This dramatic transformation of motor abilities occurs automatically with little notice or fanfare. Because normal motor development evolves in a predictable fashion, the changes often transpire unnoticed. Only when an infant demonstrates delayed or suspicious motor patterns are professionals asked to observe and assess infant motor skills. Assessments document abnormal tone, abnormal reflexes, and abnormal patterns of movement. However, abnormal motor development cannot be recognized and correctly interpreted without a solid knowledge of normal motor development.

Pediatric physical and occupational therapists assessing infants for deviations in motor development require an in-depth understanding and appreciation of normal motor development. A knowledge of normal motor skills enables clinicians to determine precisely why an infant is experiencing difficulty with a particular motor skill; it also often provides solutions to the problem. Normal motor development must be the reference point clinicians use to understand abnormal motor development and to formulate treatment techniques.

How do infant motor skills evolve? What are the factors influencing the rate, pattern, sequence, and quality of motor development? How does the therapist's interpretation of motor development influence the treatment of infants with motor delays? To answer these questions we must examine the theories of motor development that form the rationale for our interventions in pediatric physical and occupational therapy.

In general, a theory summarizes and explains observations; it consists of a series of statements describing the laws, principles, and beliefs associated with the observations (LeFrancois, 1982). Laws are statements whose accuracy is beyond reasonable doubt; theories of physics, chemistry, and other natural sciences are characterized by a number of laws. Beliefs are statements that are less substantiated by rigid experimental results. Applied sciences such as physical and occupational therapy rely more on beliefs to affirm their theories. Although a theory based on beliefs is not as strong as one based on laws, it is important to remember that no theory, even one structured on laws, is irrefutable. A theory permits predictions to be made concerning the behavior studied. Thus a theory of motor development predicts the patterns of emerging motor skills and attempts to provide an explanation for the behaviors observed.

In pediatric physical and occupational therapy, intervention strategies should be grounded on a theoretical framework of motor development that provides a rationale for techniques employed in the clinical setting. Treatments initiated by therapists should be based on theory; clinicians should be able to provide a theoretical justification for their clinical decision making and application of therapeutic interventions.

In this chapter, two theories of motor development are presented: the neuromaturational model and the systems approach. They are not the only theories of motor development; they were selected for discussion because they represent different theoretical perspectives of motor development. In spite of differences between these two theories, many of the clinical interventions used by pediatric therapists can be substantiated by either theoretical model. However, the rationale for the same intervention may arise from fundamentally different beliefs in each theory. Neither theory is being endorsed; they are presented so that the assumptions of each theory may be compared and contrasted.

Research in motor development has been relatively dormant over the last 40 years, and many issues remain unresolved. A recent resurgence of interest in motor development is stimulating therapists to evaluate the theoretical frameworks of motor development that govern many of their therapeutic interventions. In this spirit of questioning, issues raised in the literature concerning both theories of motor development are presented along with a discussion of the clinical implications of each model.

THE NEUROMATURATIONAL THEORETICAL MODEL

The neuromaturational theory of motor development, which is the traditional model of motor development, provides the framework for many of the treatment techniques used in physical and occupational therapy. Gesell and Amatruda (1947) and McGraw (1945) both advocated this model, and it remains the most frequently cited theory in textbooks of motor development written for physical and occupational therapists (Scherzer and Tscharnuter, 1982; Short-DeGraff, 1988).

The main tenet of the neuromaturational theory proposes that changes in gross motor skills during infancy result solely from the neurological maturation of the central nervous system (CNS). Maturation is characterized by increased myelination of the CNS and concomitant inhibition of the lower subcortical nuclei of the brain by the higher functioning cerebral cortex. This model assumes that the instructions, or "blueprint," for the emergence of motor skills is encoded, or "hardwired," in the brain. The cerebral cortex is construed as the organizational center for controlled movement. Within this model, motor development and changes in motor skills are intrinsically driven, and the impact of the environment plays a secondary role in the emergence of motor skills. At all stages of motor development, the intrinsic influence of the CNS transcends any effect the environment may contribute.

Advances in the science of embryology influenced the perspectives of both McGraw (1945) and Gesell (1945). Embryologists, using new microscopic techniques, were discovering that the embryo developed in a symmetrical manner, beginning in cephalocaudal and proximal to distal directions (Coghill, 1929). McGraw and Gesell extrapolated these findings to their observations of infant motor development. Four assumptions characterize the neuromaturational model:

1. Movement progresses from primitive, mass movement reflex patterns to voluntary, controlled movement.
2. Motor development progresses in a cephalocaudal direction.
3. Movement is first controlled proximally and then distally.
4. The sequence of motor development is consistent among infants, and the rate of motor development is consistent for each infant.

Therapists with even minimal experience in developmental pediatrics will immediately recognize the first three assumptions as the basis for various treatment approaches for motor-delayed and neurologically damaged infants. The fourth assumption is less evident but evolves from the theoretical framework of the neuromaturational model. Each of these assumptions is discussed separately.

Reflex to Voluntary Movement

Within the neuromaturational model, the neonate's movement patterns are interpreted as being initially dominated by reflexes such as the plantar and palmar grasp, the asymmetrical tonic neck reflex, primary stepping, the tonic labyrinthine reflex, the Moro reflex, and rooting. These movements operate in a stimulus-response fashion, with the appropriate stimulus eliciting a predictable, stereotyped response (Fiorentino, 1981). Primitive reflexes are assumed to represent the dominance of lower levels of the CNS—the subcortical nuclei located in the brain stem. Similarly, the integration of these early reflexes is perceived to indicate maturation of the CNS and inhibition of the lower centers by the higher functioning cerebral cortex. Viewed from this perspective, primitive reflexes offer a tangible gauge to assess the level of maturation of the CNS. As a result, evaluation and documentation of the presence or lack of primitive reflexes are used extensively in infant motor assessments to evaluate the level of neurological integrity (Capute et al., 1978; Fiorentino, 1981). The persistence of these reflexes past the accepted age of integration is interpreted as abnormal, representing a lack of maturation of the cerebral cortex and its subsequent inhibitory control over the lower centers. Movement evolves from an uncontrolled reflexive state to a controlled voluntary state as the cerebral cortex matures. Thus the refinement of movement is dependent on CNS maturation.

Development in a Cephalocaudal Direction

Using data collected from longitudinal observational studies of infants, Shirley (1931) concluded that motor development progresses in a cephalocaudal direction. An infant first gains voluntary head control, and the control of motor skills descends sequentially through the shoulder girdle, trunk, pelvis, and lower limbs. Consistent with the neuromaturational model, McGraw (1945) explained this developmental sequence in terms of cortical maturation; she postulated that cortical centers controlling head, trunk, and upper extremities mature before cortical centers controlling the pelvis and lower extremities. This theoretical assumption has influenced the treatment of infants with motor disorders; early treatment goals often include the facilitation of head and trunk control before progressing to pelvic control.

Proximal-Distal Development

In the same manner that motor skills have been hypothesized to emerge in a cephalocaudal direction, motor control has been described as proceeding in a proximal-distal direction. This hypothesis was first proposed by Irwin (1932, 1933) and later adopted by Gesell and Amatruda (1947). Thus an assumed prerequisite for the development of fine motor skills is trunk and shoulder control; similarly, pelvic control is necessary before an infant uses the lower limbs in crawling. The treatment aims of stability before mobility and proximal control before the facilitation of more distal skills are based on this concept. For example, a therapist would not expect proficiency in fine motor skills until an infant achieved stability at the trunk and shoulder girdle. A definite time sequence is implied with this assumption: proximal skills precede distal skills.

Rate and Sequence of Motor Development

Two parameters of motor development (rate and sequence) are subsumed in both the theoretical model and subsequent treatment plans. Rate refers to the period an infant requires to progress from one motor skill to another. Sequence of motor development defines the order in which motor skills emerge; that is, head control precedes rolling, sitting emerges before standing, and so on. Since the majority of studies on infant motor development have collected cross-sectional rather than longitudinal data, variations among individuals (interindividual variability) are discussed more often in developmental literature than is variation within the same infant (intraindividual variability). Although some variability of motor skills among infants is recognized, it is widely accepted that the sequence of motor skills is consistent. Although a child may miss a skill entirely, such as crawling, the other remaining skills emerge in a predicted order. Because of this predictable, sequential pattern of motor development, assessment of milestones provides an observable way to evaluate motor skills and to detect deviance or motor delay. The pattern of skills may vary across individuals, but the order remains constant for the majority of normally developing infants.

Rate of development has been well documented in various populations and has resulted in the availability of age norms for each motor skill. Examples of normative tests include the Bayley Scales of Infant Development (Bayley, 1969), the Peabody Fine and Gross Motor Scales (Folio and Fewell, 1983), and the Denver Developmental Screening Test (Frankenburg et al., 1970). Norms indicate the average age at which each motor skill emerges and are used to detect infants who demonstrate significant delays in achieving motor milestones. Age ranges for each skill acknowledge the variability among normal infants in the establishment of motor skills. Normative tests are not always in accord on the exact time span for each skill (Touwen, 1981); the age ranges may differ slightly for the same motor skill, but there is a general consensus on when major motor skills should be present.

Normative data have most often been gathered cross-sectionally, with many infants sampled at the same ages to document skills. Few infants have been followed longitudinally to record individual rates of development. As a result, information on the intraindividual variability in the rate of development is not as readily available. Do normally developing infants demonstrate a stable rate of change or can they develop motor skills slowly at one stage and accelerate the rate at another stage? Based on the neuromaturational model, the rate of change within an individual should be steady and dependent on the rate of neurological maturation. Anthropometric measures such as height, weight, and head circumference are based on a premise of a steady rate of development. If an infant's head circumference falls below its established curve, there is reason for concern. Similarly, if an infant suddenly demonstrates a delay in the developmental curve without an explanatory factor, such as illness, clinicians are concerned. Sequential follow-up examinations are conducted to ensure that an infant's motor skills are emerging in a consistent manner. If discontinuous rates of development were perceived as normal, early delays would cause less anxiety.

In summary, the neuromaturational theory of motor development is based on an intrinsically driven, maturational model controlled by the cerebral cortex. It provides the rationale for many of the therapeutic strategies used extensively by pediatric therapists. Although this is the most frequently cited theory of motor development, a review of the current literature raises some questions about the four assumptions of this traditional model of motor development.

ISSUES ARISING FROM THE NEUROMATURATIONAL MODEL

Within the framework of the neuromaturational model of motor development, reflexes are described as stereotyped responses to external stimuli, and their integration indicates inhibition of lower brain stem centers by the cerebral cortex. Touwen (1978) preferred the term *reactions* rather than reflexes and queried the stimulus-response definition. He argued that the brain is capable of spontaneously generating its own activity; therefore, reactions may not be stimuli-dependent. He also questioned the description of reflexes as being stereotyped and suggested that a normal neonate can respond to the same stimulus with a variety of motor responses. Touwen analyzed the finger movement patterns to repeated stimulation of the palmar grasp in five neonates; he reported that the sequence of finger flexion varied in three of five trials for each infant, even with standardization of body postures and the infants' state of arousal. He concluded that the early reflexes of newborns cannot be compared with the reflexes present in neurologically damaged infants and adults or with the reflexes present in decerebrate animals. The responses of healthy newborns were characterized by variability rather than stereotyped responses. This concept of normal variability of primitive reflexes is contrary to that put forward by the neuromaturational model.

The issue of integration and inhibition of reflexes by the maturing cerebral cortex has also been scrutinized. Zelazo (1983) demonstrated that primary stepping movements can be maintained with continued practice. Infants whose parents supported their bodies and stimulated stepping for 8 minutes daily retained the movement longer than did a comparison group of infants who received either passive exercise or no exercise. His results suggest that primary stepping can be retained with practice, and its disappearance is not totally dependent upon cortical maturation. Zelazo suggested that the retention of the reflex represents a learned response. Based on these infants demonstrating stepping skills before adequate trunk control had developed, Zelazo also questioned the validity of the assumption of motor development evolving in a cephalocaudal direction. He proposed that the cephalocaudal assumption may be based on cultural biases of motor development; in Western culture it is expected that infants will sit with support and grasp toys before they stand or walk. Zelazo cited studies conducted by Super (1976) with East African infants who were advanced in sitting, standing, and walking and delayed in crawling and rolling when compared with American infants. The former activities were encouraged by the infants' mothers because they led to early independence; thus child rearing practices may have an impact on motor development.

The assumption that motor development proceeds in a cephalocaudal direction has been evaluated by physical therapists (Horowitz and Sharby, 1988). Twenty full-term infants were observed once every 2 weeks from the age of 8 to 28 weeks, and the emerging extension postures of the head, upper extremities, and lower extremities were rated. The prone extension posture did not emerge in a cephalocaudal manner; extension of the head was followed by extension of the lower limbs, and then upper extremity extension. This finding is contrary to the response predicted by the neuromaturational model. To fit the assumptions of the model, extension in the prone position should emerge in sequential order, beginning with the head, then proceeding to the upper extremities, followed by the lower extremities.

Fetters and associates (1988) evaluated the relationship of proximal and distal motor control in the upper extremities. Kinematic recordings were obtained in 10 infants reaching for a cube at three points in time—at 5, 7, and 9 months of age. Proximal and distal control were rated on separate scales, and the resulting scores were correlated. Results indicated that proximal and distal control develop simultaneously, rather than sequentially as assumed in the neuromaturational model of motor development.

Although sequencing of motor skills may be linked to cultural variations, different cultural practices do not always result in a different sequence of motor skills. For example, Hopi Indian infants who were strapped onto a cradleboard for long periods during infancy did not demonstrate delays in walking independently when compared with Hopi infants who were not placed in the restraining device (Dennis and Dennis, 1940). Difficulty arises in trying to tease out the effect of cultural traditions on motor skills from the genetic component of different cultures and races. Infants from different cultures may have inherited dissimilar genetic blueprints for the sequence of emergence of motor skills. How much is influenced by child rearing practices and how much is intrinsically ordered by heredity? The question remains unanswered.

In summary, pediatric therapists are comfortable with the neuromaturational theory of motor development; we are familiar with its beliefs and its biological foundation. In addition, some of our fundamental treatment strategies are affirmed in this theory. Some discrepancies in the theory have been raised in recent studies evaluating components of motor development. If the studies demonstrate internal validity, the theory should be revisited and reevaluated.

SYSTEMS THEORY OF MOTOR DEVELOPMENT

The systems theory encompasses all areas of development and is derived from developmental psychology. Recently its principles and beliefs have been directed toward explaining motor development. The premise for the systems theory originates from theories of physics, chemistry, and mathematics. Researchers involved in the natural sciences observed that when elements of a system work together, certain behaviors or properties emerge that cannot be predicted from the elements separately. A new behavior is constructed, which is dependent on the input of all the contributors in the system. This behavior may have characteristics that could not have been determined by evaluating the contributing behaviors individually (Thelen et al., 1987).

This observation was extrapolated to human movement by Bernstein (1967), a Soviet neurophysiologist. He observed that joints and muscles never work in isolation but rather in coordinated patterns. Muscle synergies are a familiar concept for clinicians using the exercise techniques of proprioceptive neuromuscular facilitation, in which muscles are strengthened and recruited in functional patterns rather than individually. Bernstein postulated that the brain controls muscle groups rather than individual units. He further suggested that the muscle synergy itself is able to autonomously modify a movement independent of, or at least not totally controlled by, higher centers of the CNS. That is, a group of muscles, bones, and tendons can modulate a motor behavior without receiving instructions from the cerebral cortex. This concept is in contrast to the hierarchical, intrinsically driven structure of the neuromaturational model.

The neuromaturational theory of development evolved from a prescriptive, structural framework in which the instructions controlling movement exist before the motor behavior emerges. The instructions are encoded in the CNS, and the higher centers control movement by a "feedback" system; all modifications to a movement must originate from the cerebral cortex—the command center. In contrast, the systems approach is developed from a functional rather than a structural framework. Within this framework, the behavior itself can affect and modify the resultant behavior in contrast to all the commands being issued by the cerebral cortex. This model exemplifies a "feedforward system" that is self-correcting en route rather than hardwired from the cerebral cortex. It also implies that all factors contributing to the motor behavior are important and exert an influence on the outcome. Both of these assumptions are implicit in the dynamic motor theory arising from the systems structure (Thelen, 1987).

A practical example may help to illustrate the differences between the systems approach and the neuromaturational approach to motor development. The mastery of reaching for and grasping a toy is regarded as an important infant motor skill. In the neuromaturational model, this skill would be explained by inhibition of the primitive reflexes, trunk and head control, and proximal stability providing the basis for the distal fine motor skill of grasping. All these subsets of the skill have been orchestrated by the cerebral cortex and are dependent on the degree of CNS maturation. In short, an infant attempts to reach for a toy when neurologically ready.

The dynamic motor theory also recognizes the maturational level of the CNS as an important component for success of the task, but it is not the only factor. Other variables influencing the final motor behavior include the emotional state of the infant, the degree of motivation, cognitive awareness, the infant's posture while attempting to reach, muscle strength, and biomechanical leverages. The shape, size, and weight of the toy also determine how the motor skill is executed. The properties of the toy represent part of the task and play a critical role in determining the type of grasp the infant will choose, the position the arm takes to assure stability, and the trajectory path of the reach. All of these components compose the system required for reaching for a toy. Each factor contributes to the movement pattern the infant uses to pick up the toy. A change in any one of the factors may modify the motor strategy used for reaching and grasping. In contrast to the neuromaturational model that recognizes only the influence of the cerebral cortex, the systems or dynamic motor theory approach takes into consideration all of the factors impinging on the motor outcome. All factors are essential to the motor system, which is a cooperative unit changing and refashioning the outcome as circumstances alter.

The following assumptions define the systems or dynamic motor theory; many of them have been discussed and illustrated in the preceding example.

Motor Behaviors Are a Product of All Contributing Subsystems

A specific motor behavior cannot be explained by only one factor; all subsystems have an impact on the behavior and influence the eventual outcome. This concept of the integration of subsystems may seem obscure, but it is paramount to the systems approach to motor development. For example, sensory and motor influences cannot be separated in the systems approach. In the neuromaturational model, afferent impulses are assumed to be sensory and efferent pathways motor in nature. In the systems model, sensory and motor inputs are not identified as separate entities but rather as one system having an impact on both input and output (Reed, 1982). Sensory pathways do not transmit information to the brain, where it is received, acted upon, and sent out as a motor component. Rather, sensory and motor influences work together nested within each other, simultaneously filtering, assessing input, and contributing to the output. Afferent and efferent pathways are made up of both sensory and motor components and cannot be partitioned into separate compartments.

Movements Are Influenced by the Task

In addition to the many internal subsystems contributing to the behavior, the task influences the motor behavior. The same motor skill may be performed in more than one way, depending on the constraints imposed by the task itself. In the reaching example, the physical characteristics of the toy supply the task constraints and help determine the reaching and grasping strategies employed by the infant. Thus the task merges as an integral component of the system.

Systems Exhibit Self-Organizing, Autonomous Properties

Bernstein (1967) contended that all motor behaviors are not intrinsically driven by the CNS in a feedback manner. Within the system, motor behavior can be modulated by other mechanisms. For this to occur there must be horizontal motor control mechanisms in addition to the vertical pathways terminating in the cerebral cortex. The vertical ascending pathway may provide minimal instructions to regulate or initiate the capabilities of the system, but fine tuning and corrections can be made by mechanisms other than those initiated in the cerebral cortex. Examples of these mechanisms include muscle synergies, joints, ligaments, and lower motor neuron synapses.

Subsystems May Develop Asynchronously

The factors influencing and changing a motor behavior may not change or develop at the same rate. As a result, any one of the factors may become "rate-limiting," preventing the system from generating a specific motor behavior. Thelen and Fisher (1982) have discussed the concept of rate-limiting factors thoroughly in their investigations of primary stepping in infants. They questioned the accepted explanation that primary stepping disappears because of inhibition of lower centers in the CNS. Rather they attributed the disappearance of primary stepping to biomechanical factors, specifically an increase in fat tissue in infants during the first few months of life. The increase in adipose tissue disrupts the fat:muscle ratio; thus, the infant lacks the strength to continue stepping when held upright. This hypothesis was substantiated in a further study: manipulation of leg mass by the addition of weights inhibited stepping, whereas submersion in water facilitated stepping movements (Thelen et al., 1984). These results suggest that biomechanical factors can limit a behavior. Other factors present in a system can also be viewed as rate-limiting; a mentally handicapped infant demonstrating motor delays is an example familiar to pediatric therapists.

All four of these principles are part of the systems motor theory. Systems are complex, synthesized structures composed of the infant, the environment, and the targeted task. Each of these three components contributes to the eventual motor behavior, and the system can initiate changes in a motor behavior independent of cerebral cortex control. The system also is self-regulating and exerts limits on its motor repertoire. What are the factors or constraints that either limit or change motor behaviors?

Three different levels of constraints have been identified (Newell, 1985). Although they are discussed separately, they should not be viewed as autonomous in keeping with the premise that synthesis and interaction among factors produce behavior. Rather, consider them nesting or spiraling within each other, yielding a combined effect on motor development.

Organismic Constraints

Limitations imposed on motor behaviors by the physical and neurological characteristics of the infant are organismic constraints. This category includes the maturation of the CNS, biomechanical forces, muscle strength, disproportionate head size, trunk:limb ratios, and so on. The organismic constraint receiving most attention in the treatment of infants with neurological dysfunction is the integrity of the CNS; less frequently, other biomechanical constraints are considered. This emphasis is justifiable because neurological damage represents a critical rate-limiting factor. However, other organismic constraints may be more responsive to intervention and should also be addressed.

Environmental Constraints

Environmental factors not related to a specific task make up this category of constraints, with the most obvious member of this group of constraints being gravity. Gravity has an impact on an infant's development from the moment of birth, and all movement during the first year of life involves gaining greater control against gravity. Increasing postural control permits an infant to overcome the forces of gravity; thus lack of postural control can be viewed as a rate-limiting factor preventing the appearance of more mature motor skills. The "liberated movement activities" of Amiel-Tison and Grenier (1986) support this premise. Using this technique, an infant's lack of head control is compensated for by manual support of the head. Under the influence of this artificial postural control, more mature skills emerge; very young infants attempt to reach and grasp, and lateral righting reactions are evident. From these results it can be argued that these motor capabilities are present at birth, but because of gravitational force they do not emerge until postural control has matured to counteract gravity's influence.

Although gravity is the most obvious environmental constraint, other factors should be considered. The temperature of the surroundings, restrictive clothing, the noise level, and lighting are examples of other environmental factors that may affect an infant's motor behaviors.

Task Constraints

The restrictions on motor behavior imposed by the nature of the task are referred to as task restraints. Established motor behaviors may be altered for specific tasks. For example, mature walking in a toddler often regresses to an immature, wide-based pattern if the task is to walk on an uneven surface. When faced with the task of crawling on rough terrain, many infants alter their motor behavior by extending their knees and "bear-walking." The unique features of each of these tasks (uneven surface and rough terrain) have shaped the infant's motor behavior. With an emphasis on function, occupational therapists have been more sensitive to the importance of task constraints. It is an area that deserves more attention and has many implications for treatment.

In summary, the systems approach to motor development represents a holistic model. The infant, the environment, and the functional significance of the task cannot be isolated from each other. They represent a synthesized unit, and the motor behavior observed as an output is a product of their interactions. The system is capable of autonomously modifying the motor skill, depending on the constraints imposed on the system and the level of functioning of each unit in the system. Elements composing the system may mature at different rates, and any factor can act as rate-limiting, delaying the emergence of a new skill. With the influence of so many agents on any motor skill, the systems approach challenges the clinician to assess and evaluate infants exhibiting motor delays using a different strategy than the traditional neuromaturational assessment. What are the implications of the two theories for clinical intervention?

THEORETICAL IMPLICATIONS FOR TREATMENT

Fundamental treatment principles appear to be embedded in the neuromaturational model of motor development. The emergence of motor skills in cephalocaudal and proximal-distal directions and the refinement from reflexive to voluntary movements are all beliefs incorporated into the planning of intervention strategies with motor-delayed infants. Therapists attempt to inhibit the influence of the asymmetrical tonic neck reflex by encouraging symmetrical postures. Head control is facilitated before pelvic control, and proximal stability is achieved before distal mobility is anticipated. These principles dominate the neuromaturational model of motor development; accordingly, this theory of motor development provides the framework and basis for many of our treatment strategies.

Unfortunately, a critical limitation exists in adopting this theory of motor development as the foundation for therapeutic treatment principles. Within the neuromaturational model, all changes in motor behavior are viewed as intrinsically driven; the environment has a minimal impact on evolving motor skills. The rate, quality, and sequence of motor skills are genetically predetermined. Since treatment represents a form of environmental manipulation, it cannot be assumed from the neuromaturational model that treatment is capable of either changing a motor behavior or having an impact on the CNS. It is contrary to the neuromaturational model to surmise that damage to the cerebral cortex can be modified by external factors. Yet this is precisely what therapy advocates; motor output can be influenced by more normal sensory and motor cue input.

Even though the developmental scheme of motor skill development present in the neuromaturational model comprises the sequence of motor development familiar to therapists, this theory does not provide a rationale for intervention. In fact, intervention is the antithesis of the hierarchical, cerebral cortex–dominated framework associated with the neuromaturational model. All change must be initiated from the cerebral cortex. Although many of our beliefs concerning motor development are present in the model, the specific rationale for treatment is not. Other theories, particularly those discussing brain plasticity (Bishop, 1982), may support treatment but they do not include descriptions of the evolution of motor skills in infants. Thus, no single theory embraces both our beliefs concerning the emergence of motor skills and a rationale for treatment. Therapists must be aware of this limitation; it challenges us to search for other theories to provide support for treatment techniques used in infants with motor disorders.

The systems theory of motor development embraces the role of intervention; in fact, one weakness of the model is that no designated boundaries defining treatment exist. Because of the influence of many subsystems, and because the cerebral cortex is not viewed as the control center, many opportunities exist to facilitate motor behaviors. For example, changing an infant's posture from extension to flexion helps to overcome the environmental constraint of gravity and allows the infant to interact more effectively with the task presented. Positioning and seating in older children can also be viewed as maximizing their postural control and allowing optimum intervention with the environment. Therapists currently employ both of these treatment procedures, but they are based on the belief that positioning will inhibit tone rather than have an impact on an environmental constraint. The systems approach challenges clinicians to reinterpret why treatment techniques are effective.

The integration of the many factors influencing the emergence of motor skills opens new possibilities for treatment techniques. Awareness of the strengths and weaknesses of all subsystems in a motor-delayed infant may suggest different treatment strategies. Physical and occupational therapists have spent a great deal of time and effort helping children with cerebral palsy overcome the constraints imposed by gravity, but in the process they may have neglected other parameters. With careful assessment of all aspects of an infant's capabilities and rate-limiting factors, a more comprehensive treatment approach could be implemented, using all the positive attributes the infant possesses. Motor skills cannot be separated from an infant's other interactions with the environment; all subsystems contribute to the enhancement or delay of motor behaviors. Palmer and coworkers (1988) found that infants with cerebral palsy participating in a stimulation program achieved higher motor scores than a comparable group of infants receiving only physical therapy. This finding might be explained by the fact that the treatment of the infants in the stimulation group focused on all of the systems rather than only the motor system.

Questions remain. What degree of deprivation in any subsystem can be compensated for by the other systems? Are some subsystems more important than others or is the severity of involvement the restricting factor? An infant with extensive neurological impairment may not develop normal motor skills even with massive stimulation of the other parameters. However, can other subsystems compensate for the neurological damage present in a child with minimal brain dysfunction, for example, attention deficit disorder? Similarly, an infant with mild social deprivation may exhibit normal motor abilities; it may take massive deprivation to affect the balance of systems. These observations suggest that humans are resilient to minor disturbances within any subsystem. The degree of resiliency is unknown; research is needed to identify the children most likely to benefit from intervention.

New challenges for intervention techniques are presented to therapists by the systems theory of motor development. However, they are not without a price. The eclectic, open-ended nature of the model presents problems for research, especially regarding efficacy issues. Many factors may have an impact on any one behavior, rendering it difficult to identify a cause and effect relationship independent of numerous intervening variables. Spurious relationships abound. Pediatric therapists have long claimed that no two children with a diagnosis of cerebral palsy are alike; the systems approach suggests that no two treatment approaches should be alike. If treatment strategies become more personalized to the needs of individual infants, it will become more difficult to evaluate the effectiveness of any one treatment program.

CONCLUSIONS

Two models of motor development have been presented, one traditional and the other contemporary. We have concluded that although the neuromaturational model contains the sequence of motor development familiar to therapists, it does not provide a sound theoretical basis for treatment. In contrast, the systems approach does not provide motor milestone guidelines but encourages therapists to broaden their treatment strategies by assessing parameters other than the CNS. Strengths and weaknesses are evident in both models. The task of the therapist is to be knowledgeable about these models and others in order to identify a theoretical basis for treatment interventions.

References

Amiel-Tison C, Grenier A: *Neurological Assessment During the First Year of Life.* New York, Oxford University Press, 1986.

Bayley N: *Bayley Scales of Infant Development.* New York, Psychological Corporation, 1969.

Bernstein N: *The Coordination and Regulation of Movement.* London, Pergamon, 1967.

Bishop B: Neural plasticity. Part 2. Postnatal maturation and function-induced plasticity. Phys Ther 1982; 62:1132–1143.

Capute AJ, Accardo PJ, Vining EPG, et al.: *Primitive Reflex Profile.* Monographs in Developmental Pediatrics, vol 1. Baltimore, University Park Press, 1978.

Coghill GE: *Anatomy and the Problem of Behavior.* New York, Cambridge University Press, 1929.

Dennis W, Dennis MG: The effect of cradling practices upon the onset of walking in Hopi children. J Gen Psychol 1940; 56:77–87.

Fetters L, Fernandez B, Cermak S: The relationship of proximal and distal components in the development of reaching. Phys Ther 1988; 68:839.

Fiorentino MR: *A Basis for Sensorimotor Development—Normal and Abnormal.* Springfield, Charles C Thomas, 1981.

Folio RM, Fewell RR: *Peabody Developmental Motor Scales and Activity Cards: A Manual.* Allen, TX, DLM Teaching Resources, 1983.

Frankenburg WK, Dodds JB, Fandal A: *Denver Developmental Screening Test: Manual* (revised ed). Denver, University of Colorado Medical Center, 1970.

Gesell A: *The Embryology of Behavior, The Beginnings of the Human Mind.* New York, Harper and Brothers, 1945.

Gesell A, Amatruda C: *Developmental Diagnosis,* 2nd ed. New York, Harper & Row, 1947.

Horowitz L, Sharby N: Development of prone extension postures in healthy infants. Phys Ther 1988; 68:32–39.

Irwin OC: The organismic hypothesis and differentiation of behavior. II. The differentiation of human behavior. Psychol Rev 1932; 39:387–393.

Irwin OC: Proximodistal differentiation of limbs in young organisms. Psychol Rev 1933; 40:467–477.

LeFrancois GR: *Psychological Theories and Human Learning.* Monterey CA, Brooks/Cole Publishing, 1982.

McGraw M: *The Neuromuscular Maturation of the Human Infant.* New York, Macmillan, 1945.

Newell KM: Constraints on the development of coordination. In: Wade MG, Whiting HTA (eds): *Motor Development in Children: Aspects of Coordination and Control.* Dordrecht, Martinus Nijhoff, 1985, pp 341–360.

Palmer FB, Shapiro BK, Wachtel RC, et al.: The effects of physical therapy on cerebral palsy: a controlled trial in infants with spastic diplegia. N Engl J Med 1988; 318:803–808.

Reed ES: An outline of a theory of action systems. J Motor Behav 1982; 14:98–134.

Scherzer AL, Tscharnuter I: *Early Diagnosis and Therapy in Cerebral Palsy.* New York, Marcel Dekker, 1982.

Shirley MM: *The First Two Years: A Study of Twenty-Five Babies.* Minneapolis, University of Minnesota Press, 1931.

Short-DeGraff MA: *Human Development for Occupational and Physical Therapists.* Baltimore, Williams & Wilkins, 1988, pp 449–459.

Super CM: Environmental effects on motor development: the case of African precocity. Dev Med Child Neurol 1976; 18:561–567.

Thelen E: The role of motor development in developmental psychology: a view of the past and an agenda for the future. In: Eisenber N (ed): *Contemporary Topics in Developmental Psychology.* New York, Wiley, 1987, pp 3–33.

Thelen E, Fisher DM: Newborn stepping: an explanation for a "disappearing reflex." Dev Psychol 1982; 18:760–775.

Thelen E, Fisher DM, Ridley-Johnson R: Shifting patterns of bilateral coordination and lateral dominance in the leg movements of young infants. Dev Psychobiol 1984; 16:29–46.

Thelen E, Kelso JAS, Fogel A: Self-organizing systems and infant motor development. Dev Rev 1987; 7:39–65.

Touwen BCL: Variability and stereotypy in normal and deviant development. In: Apley J (ed): *Care of the Handicapped Child.* Clinics in Developmental Medicine, No. 67. Philadelphia, JB Lippincott, 1978, pp 99–110.

Touwen BCL: The neurological development of the infant. In: Davis JA, Sobbring J (eds): *Scientific Foundations of Paediatrics,* 2nd ed. London, Heinemann Medical Books, 1981, pp 830–841.

Zelazo PR: The development of walking: new findings and old assumptions. J Motor Behav 1983; 15:99–137.

MOTOR ASSESSMENT OF THE DEVELOPING INFANT

MOTOR ASSESSMENT IN INFANTS COMPARED WITH MOTOR ASSESSMENT IN OLDER CHILDREN AND ADULTS

The motor assessment of the developing infant presents new challenges for physical and occupational therapists. Although the assessment of motor performance and deviations in that performance has always been an integral part of the practice of physical and occupational therapy, the evaluation of the motor skills of a developing infant requires an orientation to motor performance different from that normally applied to older children and adults. Specifically, the motor assessment of the developing infant entails the evaluation of an evolutionary process or maturation of motor behaviors over time. This unique emphasis on process and maturation differentiates infant motor assessment from the motor assessment of older children and adults. In the latter case, therapists are trained to evaluate an individual's motor performance in terms of skill—that is, how the individual currently is or is not able to move in relation to a previously acquired motor skill. Therapy interventions involve helping individuals regain mastery of the performance of everyday tasks. The underlying assumption in both the assessment and treatment of motor disorders is that a normal motor pattern has been impaired or replaced with an abnormal pattern of movement; thus, the assessment and resulting treatment are aimed at assisting the individual to overcome the deficiencies of movement by relearning motor programs of performance (Gentile, 1987).

The assessment of motor performance in older children and adults with motor impairments is based not only on a physical evaluation of certain parameters, such as muscle strength and tone, range of motion, and coordination, but also on an implicit understanding of the impairment and its pathophysiology. The underlying premise has been that an individual was able to move "normally" until affected by the impairment in question. It is also generally assumed that there is a direct relationship between the anatomical impairment and function. For example, spinal injuries have traditionally been categorized on the basis of the location of the lesion so that C5, T12, and L1, for example, denote the point of the injury. This classification system has guided the assessment and treatment of individuals with spinal cord injuries (Davis and Rizzo, 1991).

The reliance on an impairment model has spawned a variety of assessment tools that emphasize the impact of the specific impairment on motor performance. For example, the motor assessment of an individual with an impairment to the central nervous system (CNS) often focuses on the effects of the impairment, such as the testing of reflex responses and stereotyped patterns of posture and movement. As a result of this conceptual framework, physical and occupational therapy assessments of motor performance have been largely restricted to the evaluation of the deviations in movement that have resulted from specific physiological or biomechanical impairments.

In addition, evaluations based on the impairment model often emphasize the assessment of abilities or skills at a specific point in time—a static "outcome" of an impairment—rather than the assessment of an ongoing developmental "process." Within this framework, the assessment of a specific skill is just that, a judgment about how the individual moves or does not move at that point in time. The movement or skill is defined according to how the individual used to perform it, and the deficiencies in the impaired movement often dictate the focus of both the assessment and the treatment procedures.

The emphasis of the assessment is often to identify the missing attributes of the movement, that is, muscle weakness or atrophy, limited range of motion, or compensatory movements, rather than the positive attributes or strengths of the movements. This approach, although perhaps appropriate for individuals who have lost a previously acquired motor skill, needs to also include an evaluation of the strengths of the observed movements when assessing evolving motor behaviors in infants.

Over the past 10 to 15 years, this classic framework of motor assessment has been expanded to include the assessment of motor performance in the developing infant. This expansion has been largely the result of a concomitant change in the survival rates of infants at extreme risk for CNS damage and a heightened appreciation for the potential role of early intervention in minimizing the effects of a CNS insult. Because of their expertise in motor assessment, therapists have been called upon to evaluate these young survivors and make recommendations about their care and management.

Motor assessments of young infants are usually performed to meet one of two objectives: (1) identification and classification or (2) programming for intervention and remediation (King-Thomas, 1987). At present, physical and occupational therapists are assessing infants in numerous milieus in order to meet one or both of the objectives.

This increased demand for the assessment of developing motor skills has required that the definition of motor performance be broadened to include the process or developmental component, in addition to the outcome or skill component. McGraw (1945) defined motor development as the sequential change in specific motor activities with age, thereby often referring to it as *motor maturation*. Accordingly, the motor skills of the developing infant are not static but rather, at any one point in time, represent an interim stage of a complex evolutionary process. Indeed, most of the skills evaluated during the first year of life are discarded by the time the infant celebrates the first birthday; thus, as isolated individual motor skills they are insignificant and only gain in importance because they provide valuable information about the overall process of motor development. For this reason, the motor assessment of the developing infant must acknowledge the dynamic nature of the motor skills being evaluated and incorporate the concept that the assessment is evaluating a process as well as specific outcomes.

In addition, the motor assessment of the developing infant is not based on an impairment or medical model. Therapists are being asked to assess infants who are at risk for motor disorders and who have not yet been diagnosed with any specific impairment or disability. Indeed, the large majority of infants who are assessed will be found to be developing normally. Even some of the infants who are known to have specific CNS lesions may defy expectations and develop a normal repertoire of movements (Vohr et al., 1989). For this reason, the pathophysiology of a specific impairment is less important to the assessment of infants who are at risk than it is to the assessment of children who have a diagnosed motor disorder. Clearly, at-risk infants represent a new group of infants with different assessment needs than those previously identified as infants with specific motor impairments or disorders.

In addition, therapists are expected to identify the infant's positive attributes of movement, rather than only the shortcomings or limitations in motor performance. The challenge for pediatric therapists is, therefore, to understand and evaluate how motor skills mature and evolve in the developing infant, regardless of the impairment the infant may or may not have. The therapist can use neither the infant's previous motor performance nor the expected deficiencies associated with a specific insult as a guide; instead one must possess a thorough understanding of the dynamics of normal motor development and the ability to observe and quantify one's findings. Therapists need to know what motor skills the infant performs and how can they be improved.

In summary, the motor assessment of the developing infant differs from other motor assessment paradigms because of its conceptual framework, its emphasis on process rather than outcome, its disregard for the medical impairment or diagnosis, and its concern for the identification of the positive attributes rather than the shortcomings of movement. These distinctions require that therapists use modified skills and approaches when assessing motor development in infancy.

BACKGROUND

Physical and occupational therapists are increasingly being called upon to assess infants who are at risk for CNS dysfunction. Graduates of neonatal intensive care units (NICUs) who either weighed less than 1500 g at birth or experienced other adverse perinatal events, such as hypoxic ischemic encephalopathy, bronchopulmonary dysplasia, or bacterial meningitis, are considered to be at increased risk for developmental problems, with motor delays accounting for the largest proportion of these problems (Coolman et al., 1985; Saigal et al., 1982). Neonatal follow-up programs have been established to monitor the development of these at-risk infants.

The major objective of these follow-up programs is the identification of developmental delays as early as possible in an infant's life. Because of the dramatic transformation in observable motor skills during the first 18 months of life, developmental experts often rely on the assessment of motor capabilities to provide them with early clues as to the overall developmental integrity of the infant. It is widely acknowledged that motor development is one of the best indicators of developmental well-being in the first year of life (Scherzer and Tscharnuter, 1990). Given their well-recognized expertise in motor development, physical and occupational therapists are participating in these follow-up programs to assess the motor maturation of at-risk infants.

Once identified, infants with signs of motor dysfunction are generally referred for early physical and occupational therapy aimed at remediating or minimizing the infant's motor problems. Recent estimates suggest that 10 to 15% of at-risk NICU survivors will exhibit major disabling conditions, such as cerebral palsy, with an additional 20 to 25% manifesting more minor problems, such as perceptual-motor disorders and learning disabilities (Saigal et al., 1982; Sell, 1986; Yu et al., 1986). Clearly, the current trend in the remediation of motor dysfunction in children is early identification and treatment within the first year of life. As a result of this trend, therapists are in need of reliable and valid assessment measures of infant motor development to clinically assess infants at risk, monitor motor development over time, and evaluate the efficacy of intervention programs for at-risk infants.

ASSESSMENT TOOLS

Considerable interest has focused on the skills and capabilities of the newborn infant and the possibility of detecting deviations in these skills early in the neonatal period. As a result of this heightened concern, several instruments have been developed that assess the neurological integrity and behavioral repertoire of the newborn infant (Brazelton, 1984; Dubowitz and Dubowitz, 1981; Prechtl, 1977). Parmelee and Michaelis (1971) have identified three purposes of newborn neurological examinations: (1) the immediate diagnosis of an evident neurological problem, such as extreme hypotonia; (2) the evaluation of the day to day changes of a known neurological problem to determine the evolution of a pathological process; and (3) the long-term prognosis of a newborn who is recovering from some neonatal neurological problem or is considered at risk because of abnormalities in the pregnancy or delivery. In neonatal examinations, the appropriate reference period is limited to 38 to 42 weeks postconception, rather than measuring motor maturation over time. Indeed, these scales have limited applicability after the newborn period and are not appropriate for the assessment of the maturing infant.

Other tests have been developed to assess one aspect of early motor development, that is, the presence and evolution of primitive reflexes, such as the asymmetrical tonic neck reflex, tonic labyrinthine reflexes, and the Moro reflex (Capute et al., 1978; Milani-Comparetti and Gidoni, 1967). This mode of assessment is based on the assumption that reflexes and reactions underlie most volitional movement and that there is a relationship between functional motor achievement and reflex activity early in life (Capute et al., 1980).

Although providing information about one aspect of early motor and neurological development, these scales have little usefulness in evaluating the evolution of motor skills over time. In addition, the importance of assessing the reflex capabilities of an infant is continually being questioned because it involves the manipulation of the infant in an arbitrary fashion and provides very little information on the development of functional motor skills (Horak, 1991). Although pediatric therapists traditionally have relied on this form of assessment to provide them with information about the integrity of the CNS, there is a growing realization that additional information is required to assess and monitor the ongoing motor development of the current graduates of neonatal intensive care (Piper, 1993). Indeed, the study of spontaneous motor behavior in infants has become of increasing interest to therapists. Spontaneous, nonreflexive behaviors, previously excluded from study, are now believed to be a more accurate portrayal of an infant's abilities than are reflex responses (VanSant, 1987).

The few measures of infant motor maturation that do exist have been developed by psychologists or educators to measure motor development in terms of motor milestone acquisition only (Bayley, 1969; Folio and Dubose, 1974; Griffiths, 1954; Wolanski and Zdanska-Brincken, 1973). These scales describe motor development in a very simplistic fashion, assessing gross motor skills as the performance of an act such as rolling over, sitting alone, or walking. No attention is given to the evolutionary nature of these specific acts in terms of the variety and multitude of motor skills contributing to an infant's motor repertoire or the essential components contributing to the specific skill.

The most popular measures of infant motor development currently employed in North America are the *motor scale* of the Bayley Scales of Infant Development (BSID) (Bayley, 1969) and the *gross motor scale* of the Peabody Developmental Motor Scales (PDMS) (Folio and Fewell, 1983). Although these two scales are widely used because of acceptable indices of reliability, neither scale evaluates motor development according to the parameters typically appraised by therapists.

The *motor scale* of the BSID contains an uneven distribution and insufficient number of items to adequately evaluate motor skills at all age levels in infancy (Ramsay and Piper, 1980). For example, at 9 months of age, there are three items, with no items at 10 months, and only two items at 11 months. Consequently, an 11-month-old infant who happens to fail the two items at 11 months of age would be assessed as functioning at the 9-month level. In addition, there are omissions in the motor developmental sequences; all methods of prewalking progression are assessed by a single item at 7 months. Finally, the *motor scale* of the BSID focuses on motor milestone acquisition in a very global manner rather than on an analysis of the various aspects of movement that contribute to the specific milestone. A typical item might be *sits alone,* with neither descriptors of the essential attributes of this milestone nor any precursor items that reflect the earlier stages of sitting behaviors. As such, infants can obtain normal Bayley scores while exhibiting atypical posture and movement (Valvano and DeGangi, 1986).

The PDMS, while containing a greater number of items for each age level, is also based on skill acquisition. Although this scale attempts to measure the emergence of new skills, it does not incorporate the aspects of movement that therapists are most interested in. As noted with the Bayley scales, some children may pass specific items yet demonstrate abnormal movement patterns indicative of neuromotor dysfunction (DeGangi, 1987). The PDMS has been identified as being more useful in the assessment of older children than in the assessment of the developing infant, since many of the early items involve placing the infant in a position and eliciting a response that may not occur spontaneously as part of the child's movement repertoire. An example of this type of item calls for the placement of the child in the supine position and then requiring the child to grab a stable chair and pull to a sitting position in order to obtain a toy (Palisano and Lydic, 1984). The appropriateness of this type of arbitrary assessment technique is questionable, as the information obtained from such an approach provides little insight into how a child normally moves.

Pediatric physical and occupational therapists view these tools as gross measures of motor performance. They believe motor development and deviations in development are better assessed through analyzing the components used to achieve motor milestones, such as the ability to shift weight, the posture assumed during the motor activity, and the progressive development of antigravity muscular control (Bly, 1983). As a result of this scarcity of tests developed specifically for the use of physical and occupational therapists in the assessment of the developing infant, therapists have recently become involved in the development of several pediatric assessment tools. These new tests will enhance the therapist's ability to objectively assess and monitor motor development in infants and young children. These new tests include the Movement Assessment of Infants (MAI) (Chandler et al., 1980), the Gross Motor Function Measure (GMFM) (Russell et al., 1989), and the Pediatric Evaluation of Disability Inventory (PEDI) (Haley et al., 1989).

Although each of these scales contributes a unique approach to pediatric motor assessment, none is focused solely on the observational assessment of the motor maturation of the developing infant. The MAI was originally developed as a screening tool to identify infants at risk for cerebral palsy, with specific criteria associated with risk points developed for 4 and 8 months of age. As a result, this screening instrument provides a risk score that by itself does not provide information about the motor performance of an infant at a specific point in time in relation to age-matched peers or the change in motor performance over time. Hence, this instrument has limited value for the practicing clinician who is performing ongoing clinical assessments of infants at various ages and who is responsible for monitoring progress in motor development within a specified period. Similarly, the MAI is not particularly well suited for research investigations evaluating the impact of specific interventions used by therapists in infants with atypical motor development.

The other two instruments, the GMFM and the PEDI, have been developed to measure gross motor function and the functional ability of children with diagnosed motor disabilities (Feldman et al., 1990; Russell et al., 1989). For example, the GMFM assesses very specific performance items, such as kicking a ball with the right foot, that are normally accomplished by 5 years of age. The PEDI assesses the functional ability of chronically ill and disabled children from 6 months through 7 years of age. Item content includes self-care, bowel and bladder control, mobility and transfers, and communication and social function. These measures were constructed to evaluate change in functional activities in infants with motor disorders, rather than to monitor infant motor maturation in normal or at-risk infants.

The majority of these assessments, developed by psychologists, neurologists, and therapists, have been based on the neuromaturational theory of development, which, as enunciated by McGraw (1945) and Gesell (1945), not only has provided the conceptual framework for many of these assessments but also has determined the content of specific items. For example, several of these tools emphasize the evaluation of the reflexes that are present in early infancy and disappear with maturation with a view toward identifying infants who either present "abnormal" reflex profiles early in life or retain their early reflexes as they age (Capute et al., 1978; Chandler et al., 1980; DeGangi et al., 1983; Fiorentino, 1981; Milani-Comparetti and Gidoni, 1967). These assessments are based on the theory that motor development is initially under the control of the lower levels of the CNS, and only with maturation does the cerebral cortex assume a role in motor development. Other scales have been based on theories that state that motor development progresses in a cephalo-caudal direction and that the sequence of progression is predictable and invariant. These tools focus primarily on specific motor milestone acquisition with little concern for the essential motor components of each milestone (Bayley, 1969; Folio and Fewell, 1983; Griffiths, 1954).

With increasing evidence that the neuromaturational theoretical constructs may be too narrow to explain all of the intricacies and various aspects of motor development, the appropriateness of not only the specific assessment tools but also the components of development they emphasize are in question (Heriza, 1991). The heightened interest in the dynamic motor theory, which states that the CNS is only one subsystem of many that dynamically interact to produce movement, suggests that a new or revised approach to infant motor assessment may be needed (Heriza, 1991).

The dynamic motor theory provides a different means of conceptualizing motor development and, hence, motor assessment. Rather than viewing motor behavior solely as the unfolding of predetermined patterns in the CNS, this perspective sees motor behavior as emerging from the dynamic cooperation of the many subsystems in a task-specific context (Heriza, 1991). The adoption of the dynamic motor theory as a basis for early physical therapy assessments in infancy is attractive because it would not only alter our approach to assessment but also would permit us to retain certain aspects of our earlier orientation. Since the maturation of the CNS is acknowledged as a contributor to motor development, infant assessments should most likely contain certain components of this theory. The challenge, therefore, is to identify those aspects of the neuromaturational theory that are valid and to expand the scope of our assessments to incorporate those identified components and the other important subsystems (Piper, 1993).

To date, no single standardized measure interprets and defines the motor maturational process in these terms. The proliferation of follow-up and treatment programs for at-risk infants underlines the need for the development of a performance-based, norm-referenced, observational measure of infant motor development that incorporates those aspects of the neuromaturational theory that are valid, as well as identifies components of other important subsystems. Pediatric therapists working in neonatal follow-up and treatment programs for at-risk infants are hampered by the lack of a reliable and valid measure of motor development that assesses the aspects of motor development most often evaluated by therapists. The need for such a tool, developed by therapists for therapists, is widely acknowledged (Campbell, 1989). Until pediatric therapists have such a tool, they not only risk the misidentification and misclassification of infants but also are unlikely to unequivocally demonstrate the effectiveness of the interventions designed for and applied to at-risk infants.

One of the goals of particular interest to physical and occupational therapists is the early identification of neuromotor deficits. Only through early identification can early developmental therapy be initiated. The greatest opportunity to effect change in movement patterns may lie in the early treatment of infants with mild to moderate involvement—yet these are the children who are the most difficult to identify reliably at an early age. Clearly, the early detection of infants experiencing subtle delays in motor maturation is compromised by only monitoring motor milestones in the traditional sense as defined by the currently available instruments. Data that have been generated using these measures suggest that infants with CNS dysfunction often remain undetected until the end of the first year of life when they have failed to sit or walk independently (Bennett et al., 1981). Many therapists suggest that such "late" identification of delays impedes their ability to significantly affect the motor development of these infants because the greater part of motor maturation has already occurred.

In addition, efforts to evaluate the efficacy of physical and occupational therapy programs for at-risk infants are seriously deterred because of the lack of appropriate, standardized measures of early motor development. The results of earlier investigations on the effects of early physical therapy on the at-risk or involved infant have been criticized because of the reliance on psychomotor and neurological measures that assessed either the quantitative acquisition of motor milestones or the neurological status of the infant (Bax, 1986; Palmer et al., 1988; Piper et al., 1986). Until a maturational measure is developed that focuses on the components of early motor development, the efficacy of these costly early motor intervention programs will remain unknown.

In summary, physical and occupational therapists are becoming increasingly involved in the evaluation and treatment of the graduates of NICUs who are known to be at increased risk for motor disorders. Because this represents a new area of motor assessment that is focused on the development of movement rather than on the loss of movement skills that had been acquired earlier in life, and because current evidence suggests that the traditional neuromaturational model may be too narrow to explain all the aspects of motor development, a new model of assessment is required. Currently, no appropriate measures of infant motor maturation exist to assist therapists in the early, accurate identification of infants who are developing normally versus those who are experiencing abnormal patterns of maturation and may require intervention. Efforts to provide efficacious services for these infants are severely limited because of the lack of an appropriate instrument to measure the effect of the therapeutic programs. Without a sensitive outcome measure, costly therapy programs aimed at enhancing the motor development of at-risk infants will remain unaccountable.

References

Bax M: Aims and outcomes of therapy for the cerebral-palsied child. Dev Med Child Neurol 1986; 28:695.

Bayley N: *Bayley Scales of Infant Development.* New York, Psychological Corporation, 1969.

Bennett FC, Chandler LS, Robinson NM, et al.: Spastic diplegia in premature infants: etiologic and diagnostic considerations. Am J Dis Child 1981; 135:732–737.

Bly L: *Components of Normal Movement During the First Year of Life and Abnormal Motor Development.* Birmingham AL, Pathway Press, 1983.

Brazelton TB: *Neonatal Behavioral Assessment Scale,* 2nd ed. Clinics in Developmental Medicine, No. 88. Philadelphia, JB Lippincott, 1984.

Campbell SK: Measurement in developmental therapy: past, present and future. In: Miller LJ (ed): *Developing Norm-Referenced Standardized Tests.* New York, Haworth Press, 1989, pp 1–13.

Capute AJ, Accardo PJ, Vining EPG, et al.: *Primitive Reflex Profile.* Monographs in Developmental Pediatrics, vol 1. Baltimore, University Park Press, 1978.

Capute AJ, Shapiro BK, Wachtel RG, et al.: Motor functions: associated primitive reflex profiles. Pediatr Res 1980; 14:431.

Chandler LS, Andrews MS, Swanson MW: *Movement Assessment of Infants: A Manual.* Rolling Bay, Washington, published by the authors, 1980.

Coolman RB, Bennett FC, Sells CJ, et al.: Neuromotor development of graduates of the neonatal intensive care unit: patterns encountered in the first two years of life. J Dev Behav Pediatr 1985; 6:327–333.

Davis WE, Rizzo TL: Issues in the classification of motor disorders. Adapted Physical Activity Q 1991; 8:280–304.

DeGangi GA: Sensorimotor tests: Peabody Developmental Motor Scales. In: King-Thomas L, Hacker BJ (eds): *A Therapist's Guide to Pediatric Assessment.* Boston, Little, Brown, 1987, pp 185–190.

DeGangi GA, Berk RA, Valvano J: Test of motor and neurological functions in high-risk infants: preliminary findings. J Dev Behav Pediatr 1983; 4:182–189.

Dubowitz L, Dubowitz V: *The Neurological Assessment of the Preterm and Full-Term Newborn Infant.* Clinics in Developmental Medicine, No. 79. Philadelphia, JB Lippincott, 1981.

Feldman AB, Haley SM, Coryell J: Concurrent and construct validity of the Pediatric Evaluation of Disability Inventory. Phys Ther 1990; 70:602–610.

Fiorentino MR: *A Basis for Sensorimotor Development: Normal and Abnormal.* Springfield IL, Charles C Thomas, 1981.

Folio MR, Dubose RF: *Peabody Motor Scales.* Nashville TN, George Peabody College of Teachers, 1974.

Folio MR, Fewell RR: *Peabody Developmental Motor Scales and Activity Cards: A Manual.* Allen, TX, DLM Teaching Resources, 1983.

Gentile AM: Skill acquisition: action, movement, and neuromotor processes. In: Carr JH, Shepherd RB (eds): *Movement Science. Foundations for Physical Therapy in Rehabilitation.* Rockville MD, Aspen Publications, 1987, pp 93–154.

Gesell A: *The Embryology of Behavior, The Beginnings of the Human Mind.* New York, Harper and Brothers, 1945.

Griffiths R: *The Abilities of Babies.* London, University of London Press, 1954.

Haley SM, Faas RM, Coster W, et al.: *Pediatric Evaluation of Disability Inventory.* Boston, New England Medical Center, 1989.

Heriza C: Motor development: traditional and contemporary theories. In: *Contemporary Management of Motor Control Problems.* Proceedings of the II STEP Conference. Alexandria VA, Foundation for Physical Therapy, 1991, pp 99–126.

Horak FB: Assumptions underlying motor control for neurologic rehabilitation. In: *Contemporary Management of Motor Control Problems.* Proceedings of the II STEP Conference. Alexandria VA, Foundation for Physical Therapy, 1991, pp 11–27.

King-Thomas L: Responsibilities of the examiner. In: King-Thomas L, Hacker BJ (eds): *A Therapist's Guide to Pediatric Assessment.* Boston, Little, Brown, 1987, pp 11–18.

McGraw MB: *The Neuromuscular Maturation of the Human Infant.* New York, Macmillan, 1945.

Milani-Comparetti AM, Gidoni EA: Routine developmental examination in normal and retarded infants. Dev Med Child Neurol 1967; 9:631–638.

Palisano RJ, Lydic JS: The Peabody Developmental Motor Scales: an analysis. Phys Occup Ther Pediatr 1984; 4:69–75.

Palmer FB, Shapiro BK, Wachtel RC, et al.: The effects of physical therapy on cerebral palsy: a controlled trial in infants with spastic diplegia. N Engl J Med 1988; 18:803–808.

Parmelee AH, Michaelis R: Neurological examination of the newborn. In: Hellmuth J (ed): *Exceptional Infant,* vol 2: Studies in Abnormalities. London, Butterworths, 1971, p 7.

Piper MC: Theoretical foundations for physical therapy assessment in early infancy. In: Wilhelm IJ (ed): *Physical Therapy Assessment in Early Infancy.* New York, Churchill Livingstone, 1993, pp 1–12.

Piper MC, Kunos I, Willis DM, et al.: Early physical therapy effects on the high-risk infant: a randomized controlled trial. Pediatrics 1986; 78:216–224.

Prechtl HFR: *Neurological Examination of the Full-Term Newborn Infant.* Clinics in Developmental Medicine, No. 63. Philadelphia, JB Lippincott, 1977.

Ramsay M, Piper MC: A comparison of two developmental scales in evaluating infants with Down syndrome. Early Hum Dev 1980; 4:89–95.

Russell DJ, Rosenbaum PL, Cadman DT, et al.: The Gross Motor Function Measure: a means to evaluate the effects of physical therapy. Dev Med Child Neurol 1989; 31:341–352.

Saigal S, Rosenbaum P, Stoskopf B, et al.: Follow-up of infants 501 to 1500 g birth weight delivered to residents of a geographically defined region with perinatal intensive care facilities. J Pediatr 1982; 100:606–613.

Scherzer AL, Tscharnuter I: *Early Diagnosis and Therapy in Cerebral Palsy: A Primer on Infant Developmental Problems,* 2nd ed. New York, Marcel Dekker, 1990.

Sell EJ: Outcome of very very low birth weight infants. Clin Perinatol 1986; 13:451–459.

Valvano J, DeGangi GA: Atypical posture and movement findings in high risk preterm infants. Phys Occup Ther Pediatr 1986; 6(2):71–81.

VanSant AF: Concepts of neural organization and movement. In: Connolly BH, Montgomery PC (eds): *Therapeutic Exercise in Developmental Disabilities* (1st ed reprint). Chattanooga, Chattanooga Corporation, 1987, pp 1–8.

Vohr BR, Garcia-Coll C, Mayfield S, et al.: Neurologic and developmental status related to the evolution of visual-motor abnormalities from birth to 2 years of age in preterm infants with intraventricular hemorrhage. J Pediatr 1989; 115:296–302.

Wolanski N, Zdanska-Brincken M: A new method for the evaluation of motor development of infants. Pol Psychol Bull 1973; 4:43–53.

Yu VYH, Wong PY, Bajuk B, et al.: Outcome of extremely-low-birth-weight infants. Br J Obstet Gynaecol 1986; 93:162–170.

three

ALBERTA INFANT MOTOR SCALE: CONSTRUCTION OF A MOTOR ASSESSMENT TOOL FOR THE DEVELOPING INFANT

The need for standardized assessment tools in the clinical practice of pediatric physical and occupational therapy has been widely acknowledged (Campbell, 1989). Physical and occupational therapists often appraise the motor performance of young infants by using either their clinical judgment, supplemented with unstandardized tests adapted for their specific clinical requirements, or assessment tools developed by other professionals.

Although clinical judgment is known to be accurate and appropriate for certain therapeutic procedures and interventions, it has also been acknowledged that clinical judgments as applied to the assessment and evaluation of individuals can be significantly enhanced through systematic, standardized measurement (Sackett et al., 1985). The reasons for the limitations of clinical judgment as applied to the assessment of patients are varied. Research suggests that the nonsystematic application of diagnostic criteria, errors of omission or commission in the gathering of clinical evidence, recording inference rather than evidence, and the bias in judgment as a result of clinical expectations all interfere with the accurate assessment of clinical conditions (Ashton et al., 1991; Campbell, 1989; Sackett et al., 1985). The use of standardized assessment tools can minimize the effects of each of these factors and thereby result in a more meaningful assessment of a child's status. For example, the directions for administering and scoring standardized tests provide specific criteria for judging the observed behaviors. Using a set testing protocol prevents errors of omission. Also, use of a standard protocol guards against biased expectations in the interpretation of the observations (Campbell, 1991).

The typical response to the lack of standardized tests in the domain of pediatric physical and occupational therapy has been either the creation of specific tools in individual pediatric facilities, tailored to meet specific clinic or program needs, or the adoption of assessment tools developed by other professional groups tangentially related to physical and occupational therapy. The former approach relies primarily on anecdotal reporting and denies therapists the opportunity to systematically and objectively record and monitor performance over time. In addition, information gathered in this manner is not comparable and hence is difficult to interpret given the lack of widely accepted psychometric test features, such as reliability and validity and normative data. Indeed, it has been demonstrated that even carefully constructed, standardized assessments are often inappropriately administered and interpreted by therapists (Lewko, 1976). Hence, the possibility of obtaining objective, reliable, and valid information on the status of a child through the use of unstandardized tools is even more remote.

The latter approach of using assessment tools that have been developed by other professionals for other purposes has been less than acceptable even when the measures are correctly administered. In the area of infant motor development, physical and occupational therapists have relied largely on assessments developed by pediatricians, neurologists, psychologists, or special educators. Although each of these professional groups contributes something significant to the care and assessment of the developing infant, none brings to infant motor assessment the unique approach associated with physical or occupational therapy evaluation. Specifically, pediatric therapists are seeking tests that (1) assess "quality" of movement, including postural alignment and control, balance, and coordination; (2) capture improvement in children who change slowly; and (3) measure functional skills (Campbell, 1991). Available motor development tests, constructed and designed by other professionals, often fail to assess these features and emphasize other components of movement or development.

This dearth of motor assessment tools has encouraged therapists to develop their own evaluative measures based on the conceptual frameworks and concepts of treatment. To date, these efforts have spawned several promising instruments that should assist therapists in the assessment of the effects of treatment of children with neurological impairment and disability. Two examples of such instruments include the Gross Motor Function Measure (Russell et al., 1989) and the Pediatric Evaluation of Disability Inventory (Haley et al., 1989). These tools have been developed specifically to assess the progress and status of children with diagnosed movement disorders such as cerebral palsy. Thus, these tools are appropriately employed with children who are known to have a motor impairment and are receiving therapy aimed at minimizing the disability arising from the impairment.

The constructs and focus of the preceding instruments differ considerably from those required to assess the developing infant who may or may not have a motor impairment. Because therapists are now assessing the motor performance of normally developing and at-risk infants, in addition to those children who have diagnosed motor impairments, they are in need of an instrument that highlights the key elements of early motor development. As physical and occupational therapists become increasingly involved in the assessment, care, and management of infants who are at risk for motor disorders but who may be developing normally, the lack of a sensitive, reliable, and valid tool to assess the motor maturation and skills of the developing infant will continue to hinder their efforts.

Therapists assessing the developing infant are seeking a scale that (1) will provide information to the clinician and parents about the motor activities the infant has mastered, those that are currently developing, and those that are not in the infant's repertoire; (2) will measure motor performance in infancy that occurs with maturation or before and after intervention; (3) will measure changes in motor performance in infancy that are quite small and thus not likely to be detected using more traditional motor measures; and (4) will be an appropriate research tool to assess the efficacy of rehabilitation programs for at-risk infants.

Given these needs, a theoretically sound, performance-based, norm-referenced test that is reliable and valid to measure motor maturation of infants from term or 40 weeks postconception to the age of independent walking was constructed. The Alberta Infant Motor Scale (AIMS) was designed to fill the gaps currently present in the area of motor assessment of the developing infant. The AIMS is an observational measure of infant motor performance incorporating the theoretical concepts of motor development most frequently identified by therapists in the assessment and management of infants with motor delays. The AIMS incorporates aspects of the neuromaturational theoretical framework with relevant attributes of the dynamic motor perspective. It assesses the infant's sequential development of motor milestones from term to independent walking in terms of the progressive development and integration of antigravity muscular control in four postural positions: prone, supine, sitting, and standing.

BACKGROUND

Physical and occupational therapists are being asked to evaluate the motor status of infants at risk for central nervous system (CNS) dysfunction in order to detect, as early as possible, any deviations from the normal pattern of motor maturation. The lack of a performance-based, standardized, norm-referenced motor assessment tool has impeded these early identification efforts. Infants with subtle motor deviations often are either missed or incorrectly labeled when the current scales are employed to assess motor maturation.

The most frequent explanation for the poor prognostic record of motor assessments is the ineffectiveness of available measurement tools to accurately discriminate normal from abnormal motor skills. Many measures designed by therapists have been poorly developed and lack validation (Benson and Clark, 1982). Motor measures developed by psychologists and educators, although psychometrically sound, have not been developed using the constructs of motor development that are important to occupational and physical therapists. As a result, the tests are mere checklists of motor development rather than assessments of the components of movement necessary to achieve specific motor skills. No motor scale to date has been constructed and norm-referenced to assess sequentially the aspects of motor development that therapists routinely evaluate clinically. In addition, no measures are available to evaluate the efficacy of therapeutic motor interventions with at-risk infants.

According to Kirshner and Guyatt (1985) measures may be used for one or more of three purposes: discrimination, prediction, and evaluation. A discriminative index distinguishes between individuals with and without a particular characteristic or function. The discrimination is based on current rather than future performance, that is, the child is currently performing at a different level from the reference group. Norm-referenced measures serve this purpose, as they categorize children by means of percentile rank scores, standard scores, or age-equivalent scores. Examples of such indices include the Bayley Scales of Infant Development (Bayley, 1969) and the Peabody Developmental Motor Scales (Folio and Fewell, 1983). Scales like these are intended to discriminate children who are developmentally normal from those who are below average or definitely abnormal in achieving motor milestones. These instruments are standardized on large populations to ensure reliability and validity.

The prediction of future performance is accomplished by a predictive index that classifies individuals into categories based on what is believed or expected will be their future status. For example, this type of scale would be required to accurately predict which neonates will later exhibit cerebral palsy. Prediction is a major purpose of the Movement Assessment of Infants which was originally designed for assessing 4-month-old infants to predict their risk of developing cerebral palsy (Chandler et al., 1980).

An evaluative index is used to measure the magnitude of change in function over time or after treatment. Such a measure should be responsive to small increments of change in motor performance, resulting from either maturation or treatment. For example, the Gross Motor Function Measure is intended for use in measuring change in children with cerebral palsy and was designed specifically to measure the outcome of physical therapy for such children (Russell et al., 1989).

Although it is clear that within the domain of infant motor measurement, therapists are in need of measures that fulfill all three purposes, it may be unrealistic to expect any one measure to suffice for all three functions. Rather, a measure must be constructed and validated according to its ultimate purpose or purposes. The AIMS was developed to fulfill two of the the preceding purposes, discrimination and evaluation. Specifically, the construction of the

AIMS was predicated upon the premise that a measure was needed first to discriminate those infants who exhibited immature and atypical infant motor development at the time of the assessment from those who exhibited "normal" performance and second to evaluate small increments in performance that occur as a result of either maturation or intervention.

The ability to predict long-term outcomes from previous performance on an infant assessment, although of interest to therapists, was not seen as a primary purpose of the AIMS. The predictive validity of infant assessment tools in a variety of domains has never been particularly impressive. This may be the result of the lack of a sensitive tool or the variety of intervening factors during the time between infancy and later childhood that may account for the change in status (Piper, 1993).

Another possible explanation for poor identification of motor dysfunction in infancy involves a primary assumption embedded in the theory of normal motor development used to develop motor scales. The use of a motor scale to predict motor dysfunction operates on the premise that delay or deviance in motor performance exhibited early in an infant's life will persist as the child ages. This assumption may be erroneous; abnormal motor skills at an early age may resolve spontaneously, just as early deviations in muscle tone resolve (Drillien, 1972). Also, some types of motor dysfunction, particularly mild and moderate cases, may not be discernible until a certain level of motor development is achieved or attempted. If either of these two possibilities is true, predictive evaluation based on infant motor performance may not be feasible, and the prediction of motor outcomes in later childhood using attainment of early motor skills as an indicator may be inappropriate. Although the AIMS might eventually be shown to be a valuable predictive motor function measure, its original primary purposes were focused on discrimination and evaluation, as already noted.

The AIMS was constructed to incorporate the components of motor development that are deemed essential to the evaluation and treatment of at-risk infants. As stated previously, the AIMS assesses motor maturation of the infant from term (40 weeks postconception) through the age of independent walking by describing this motor sequence according to the development of postural control relative to the various postural positions: prone, supine, sitting, and standing. Because most motor development measures entail considerable infant handling and because infant handling has been shown to interfere with the reliability of the measures (Haley et al., 1986; Werner and Bayley, 1966), the AIMS was designed as an observational measure.

As stated earlier, the construction of the AIMS was based on certain aspects of the neuromaturational theory and identified components of the dynamic motor theory. The AIMS acknowledges the neuromaturational model in terms of the sequencing of the individual motor items. The relatively invariant sequential appearance of motor abilities has been consistently demonstrated (Ames, 1937; Gesell and Ames, 1940; McGraw, 1945; Shirley, 1931). Although cultural differences have been noted to exist in the evolution of motor skills (Super, 1976), North American infants have been consistently shown to develop certain motor skills before other more advanced skills. It is within this context that the AIMS reflects the neuromaturational model of motor development.

The AIMS also has attempted to reflect some of the more global aspects of the dynamic motor theory. Heriza (1991) identified three areas that should be addressed when assessing motor performance from the perspective of the dynamic motor theory: the relevant subsystems, the environment, and the task. The AIMS honors the basic principles of the dynamic motor theory in terms of the importance it places on the testing environment, the gravitational position of the infant, and the task in the assessment context.

Infants are to be assessed through observation in an unobtrusive environment, with minimal handling and no arbitrary stimuli or facilitation. Indeed, infants are observed as they move freely during the assessment, motivated by their environmental surroundings with no constraints imposed by the therapist. Parents are encouraged to stay close to the infant throughout the assessment; conversely, the therapist need not be within close proximity of the child during the assessment. The infant sets the pace and momentum of the assessment, with the therapist responding to the infant's cues rather than the infant being asked to respond to conditions imposed by the therapist. For example, the assessment is interrupted if the infant is anxious and is resumed only when the infant is composed. Similarly, the infant may be redressed if he or she becomes distraught or unhappy during the assessment. Functional movement, within a task context determined by the infant's interest in the surroundings, is used as the basis of assessment; the infant's own toys may be used as motivators for movement. No specific toys, prompts, or conditions are required to assess movement. In addition, the infant is assessed in four positional planes in order to evaluate movement patterns and skills in different gravitational situations.

CONSTRUCTION OF THE AIMS

The construction of the AIMS was initiated by a literature review of existing instruments and descriptive narratives of early motor development with the view to describing the functional sequences and variations that occur in early motor development (Amiel-Tison and Grenier, 1986; Bly, 1980; Saint-Anne Dargassies, 1986; Tscharnuter, 1982). Eighty-four items were generated based upon these published descriptive narratives of early motor performance. Four separate sets of items were written, corresponding to the four positions in which infants are to be assessed: prone, supine, sitting, and standing. An artist was hired to capture each item in a visual form. Each item consists of an artist's drawing of an infant in a particular position accompanied by a detailed description of the weight bearing, posture, and antigravity movements observed in that position (see chart at end of chapter).

Meetings were held with pediatric physical therapists in the province of Alberta to review the 84 items for appropriateness, content, and clinical importance. In addition, a mail inquiry was conducted of 291 members of the Pediatric Division of the Canadian Physiotherapy Association. Members were randomly sent copies of the prone items, the standing items, or the supine and sitting items. Each therapist was asked to rate the items as to their importance to motor development, the likelihood that the child would elicit that behavior during assessment, and the observability of the behavior, if elicited. In addition, they were asked to sort the items within each positional set as to their typical order of emergence and to give an age range within which each behavior should emerge in normal infants. The analyses of these responses resulted in the elimination of 17 items and the revision of certain others.

Initial placement (scaling) of the remaining items along the continuum of motor development was accomplished using the therapists' averaged estimate of the ages of emergence in normal infants. In addition, the data from the item sorting task were subjected to a multidimensional scaling procedure to assess whether dimensions other than developmental sequencing were necessary to account for the therapists' responses. Only one dimension, motor maturation, appeared necessary to account for the judgments.

Six international experts in infant motor development attended a 2-day work session as part of the content validation process. The work session was comprised of four stages. First, the experts were each given a copy of the item sets and were asked to review them independently for clarity, significance, order, and inclusiveness. Second, the six experts were divided into two groups of three members each and asked to review in detail specific item sets. Each group was (1) to determine the accurate sequence of the items within the set, (2) to remove inappropriate items from the set, and (3) to add items, if necessary, to the set. The third stage involved combining the four sets of items on a maturational continuum. The experts were then asked to review the entire set of items for redundancies, sequencing of occurrence, and omissions. Finally, a group session was held to discuss administration and scoring issues in general.

The scale was then revised and administrative guidelines were developed in light of the input received from the work session. Thirteen items were deleted and five new items were constructed, resulting in a total of 59 items. A score sheet was developed for use in a feasibility test. Three physical therapists were hired and trained in the administration of the infant motor measure in preparation of the feasibility test.

Ninety-seven low-risk infants deemed to be developing normally, who were age-stratified through the first 18 months of life, were recruited for the feasibility study through the Edmonton Board of Health well baby clinics. These infants were assessed on the infant motor maturation scale by one of the three physical therapists. The feasibility study generated recommendations concerning feasibility, the administrative guidelines, the recording form, and operational difficulties. These recommendations provided the bases for revisions of the instrument prior to reliability and validity testing.

Certain scaling models were tested on the feasibility data, including multidimensional scaling, Guttman scaling, and item response models. Although these analyses involved quite a small number of infants/age category, the items appeared to be measuring a single dimension, motor maturity, and the ordering of items on the developmental continuum was very close to what had been anticipated.

Following the collection of the feasibility data, seven items were deleted and six new items added, resulting in a total of 58 items (21 prone items, 9 supine items, 12 sitting items, and 16 standing items) to be included for the reliability and validity testing. Key descriptors that must be observed for the infant to pass each item were identified and included on the score sheets. In preparation for the reliability and validity testing, guidelines for administration and scoring were developed.

The results of the reliability and validity testing are reported in detail in Chapter 10; the procedures that were used to establish the norms for the AIMS are found in Chapter 11. Specifically, the interrater reliability, test-retest reliability, concurrent validity, and discriminative validity of the AIMS have been assessed. These tests revealed that the AIMS is extremely reliable and is valid in discriminating the motor performance of normally developing infants from that of at-risk and motoric delayed infants, and for evaluating small changes in motor skills due to maturation.

Once the AIMS was determined to be both reliable and valid, age- and sex-related norms were developed on the basis of assessing the motor performance of a cross-sectional sample of 2200 infants representative of all Albertan infants. The establishment of these norms permits the use of the AIMS as a discriminative index by providing for the identification of those infants whose performance is either delayed or aberrant in relation to their peers, or the normative group. This normative data base ensures that the performance of an individual child who is assessed with the AIMS is properly interpreted. The nature of the AIMS and the associated norms permit the administration of the scale with an infant of any age during the first 18 months of life. That is to say, therapists may use the AIMS to evaluate an infant at any point in time, from birth to 18 months of age, and interpret the scores obtained using the appropriate age norms. This is an important feature, as a wide variation currently exists in the ages of infants seen in follow-up clinics.

In summary, the AIMS represents a carefully constructed, theoretically sound, performance-based, norm-referenced, observational tool for the motor assessment of the developing infant. The 58 items of the AIMS incorporate the components of motor development that are deemed essential by therapists for the evaluation and treatment of at-risk infants. The psychometric properties of the AIMS suggest that it is a well-designed, psychometrically sound instrument, appropriate for the measurement of small increments of change in the motor development of infants. The normative data provide for the identification of those infants whose motor performance is atypical for their age. Given the widely acknowledged lack of standardized instruments for the assessment of motor development in infancy, the AIMS fills a gap in the clinical practice of pediatric physical and occupational therapy.

Prone Lying

Weight Bearing	Weight on hands, forearms, and chest
Posture	Elbows behind shoulders and close to body Hips and knees flexed
Antigravity Movement	Lifts head asymmetrically to 45° Cannot maintain head in midline

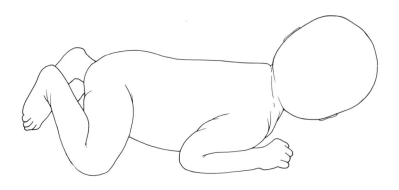

Rolling Supine to Prone Without Rotation

Weight Bearing	Weight on one side of body
Posture	Head up Trunk elongated on weight-bearing side Shoulder in line with pelvis
Antigravity Movement	Lateral head righting Rolling initiated from head, shoulder, or hip Trunk moves as one unit

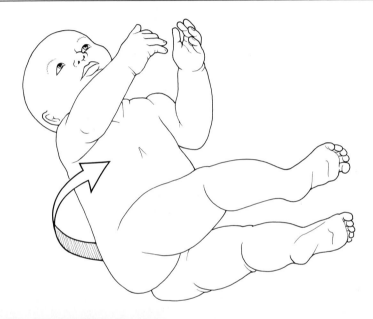

Sitting with Arm Support

Weight Bearing	Weight on buttocks, legs, and hands

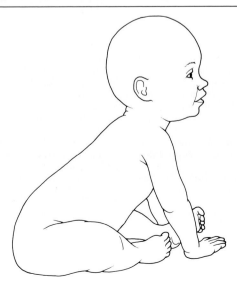

Posture	Head up; shoulders elevated Hips flexed, externally rotated, and abducted Knees flexed Lumbar and thoracic spine rounded
Antigravity Movement	Maintains head in midline Supports weight on arms briefly

Cruising Without Rotation

Weight Bearing	Weight on feet Some arm support
Posture	Legs abducted and externally rotated Wide base of support Body faces forward
Antigravity Movement	Cruises sideways without rotation

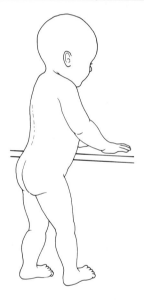

References

Ames LB: The sequential patterning of prone progression in the human infant. Gen Psychol Monogr 1937; 19:409–460.

Amiel-Tison C, Grenier A: *Neurological Assessment During the First Year of Life.* New York, Oxford University Press, 1986.

Ashton B, Piper MC, Warren S, et al.: Influence of medical history on assessment of at-risk infants. Dev Med Child Neurol 1991; 33:412–418.

Bayley N: *Bayley Scales of Infant Development.* New York, Psychological Corporation, 1969.

Benson J, Clark F: A guide for instrument development and validation. Am J Occup Ther 1982; 36:789–800.

Bly L: The components of normal movement during the first year of life. In: Slaton D (ed): *Development of Movement in Infancy.* Chapel Hill, Division of Physical Therapy, University of North Carolina, 1980, pp 85–123.

Campbell S: Measurement in developmental therapy: past, present, and future. In: Miller LJ (ed): *Developing Norm-Referenced Standardized Tests.* New York, Haworth Press, 1989, pp 1–13.

Campbell SK: Framework for the measurement of neurologic impairment and disability. In: *Contemporary Management of Motor Control Problems.* Proceedings of the II STEP Conference. Alexandria VA, Foundation for Physical Therapy, 1991, pp 143–154.

Chandler L, Andrews M, Swanson M: *Movement Assessment of Infants: A Manual.* Rolling Bay, Washington, published by the authors, 1980.

Drillien C: Abnormal neurologic signs in the first year of life in low-birthweight infants: possible prognostic significance. Dev Med Child Neurol 1972; 14:575–584.

Folio MR, Fewell RR: *Peabody Developmental Motor Scales and Activity Cards: A Manual.* Allen TX, DLM Teaching Resources, 1983.

Gesell A, Ames LB: The ontogenetic organization of prone behavior in human infancy. J Gen Psychol 1940; 56:247–263.

Haley SM, Faas RM, Coster W, et al.: *Pediatric Evaluation of Disability Inventory.* Boston, New England Medical Center, 1989.

Haley SM, Harris SR, Tada WL, et al.: Item reliability of the Movement Assessment of Infants. Phys Occup Ther Pediatr 1986; 6:21–39.

Heriza C: Motor development: traditional and contemporary theories. In: *Contemporary Management of Motor Control Problems.* Proceedings of the II STEP Conference. Alexandria VA, Foundation for Physical Therapy, 1991, pp 99–126.

Kirshner B, Guyatt G: A methodological framework for assessing health and disease. J Chron Dis 1985; 38:27–36.

Lewko JH: Current practices in evaluating motor behavior of disabled children. Am J Occup Ther 1976; 30:413–419.

McGraw MB: *The Neuromuscular Maturation of the Human Infant.* New York, Macmillan, 1945.

Piper M: Theoretical foundations for physical therapy assessment in early infancy. In: Wilhelm IJ (ed): *Physical Therapy Assessment in Early Infancy.* New York, Churchill Livingstone, 1993, pp 1–12.

Russell D, Rosenbaum PL, Cadman DT, et al.: The Gross Motor Function Measure: a means to evaluate the effects of physical therapy. Dev Med Child Neurol 1989; 31:341–352.

Sackett DL, Haynes RB, Tugwell P: *Clinical Epidemiology: A Basic Science for Clinical Medicine.* Boston, Little, Brown, 1985.

Saint-Anne Dargassies S: *The Neuro-motor and Psycho-affective Development of the Infant.* New York, Elsevier, 1986.

Shirley MM: *The First Two Years: A Study of Twenty-Five Babies.* Minneapolis, University of Minnesota Press, 1931.

Super C: Environmental effects on motor development: the case of African infant precocity. Dev Med Child Neurol 1976; 18:561–567.

Tscharnuter I: Normal and abnormal sensorimotor development. In: Scherzer AL, Tscharnuter I (eds): *Early Diagnosis and Therapy in Cerebral Palsy: A Primer on Infant Developmental Problems.* New York, Marcel Dekker, 1982, pp 73–122.

Werner EE, Bayley N: The reliability of Bayley's revised scale of mental and motor development during the first year of life. Child Dev 1966; 37:39–50.

four

ADMINISTRATION GUIDELINES

_____
_____
_____
_____
_____
_____
_____
_____
_____
_____
_____
_____
_____
_____
_____
_____
_____
_____
_____
_____
_____
_____
_____
_____
_____
_____
_____
_____
_____

AGE AND TYPE OF CLIENT

The AIMS has been constructed to measure the motor development of infants aged 0 to 18 months. The appropriate use of the AIMS within this age range is largely determined by the purpose of the particular assessment, that is, (1) the *identification* of infants who are delayed or deviant in their motor development or (2) the *evaluation* of motor development or maturation over time. If the objective of the assessment is to *identify* infants who are currently exhibiting delayed motor development, the AIMS may be used to assess all infants 18 months or younger. It is appropriate to use the AIMS to identify infants with all forms of motor delays, including those infants who are exhibiting immature motor development as well as those infants who have severe motor delays involving abnormal patterns of movement. The AIMS is only valid, however, in the identification of delays at the time of testing; the long-term predictive validity of the AIMS in identifying future delays is still unknown.

If the purpose of the assessment is to *evaluate* or monitor motor development, maturation, or change over time as the result of aging or intervention, the AIMS may be used with the following infants who are 18 months or younger: (1) infants who are exhibiting normal motor development and are being monitored over time as part of their developmental history, (2) infants who are at risk for developmental delays, (3) infants who have been diagnosed as having disorders or conditions that present with immature motor development, and (4) infants who during the course of routine well baby examinations are identified as being either immature or suspect in terms of their motor development.

The AIMS may be used to monitor the course of motor development in infants who are developing normally over the first 18 months of life. As with the well-established growth parameters, such as height and weight, the AIMS may be administered in well baby clinics to provide information to health professionals and caregivers as to the progress of the infant's motor development over time. The normative data of the AIMS permit the comparison of any infant's motor development with an age-matched peer group in terms of percentile rank. The administration of the AIMS may prove useful in providing developmental information and feedback to caregivers about the motor performance of their infants over the first 18 months of life.

Infants are considered to be at risk because of adverse genetic, prenatal, perinatal, neonatal, postnatal, or environmental influences that may lead to subsequent problems in development (Lansford, 1977). Typically, these infants have received care in a neonatal intensive care unit and are subsequently followed in neonatal follow-up clinics. The majority of these infants are born prematurely, although full-term infants with medical problems during or after birth are also included in this category. Although most of these infants develop normally, the AIMS is useful in evaluating and monitoring the motor development of at-risk infants over time in order to identify those infants who are experiencing difficulty or delays in their motor development at the time of the assessment.

The AIMS may also be used with infants who have a specific diagnosis that may include immature motor development as one of its presenting signs. Examples of such diagnoses include fetal alcohol syndrome, Down syndrome, failure to thrive, seizure disorders, bronchopulmonary dysplasia, and developmental delay. Infants with these diagnoses may exhibit hypotonia or immature or delayed acquisition of motor skills. Despite these limitations, these infants demonstrate normal patterns of movement, differentiating them from infants with more severe motor impairments who exhibit abnormal components of movement, such as infants with spina bifida or those with cerebral palsy. The AIMS may be used to assess the motor skills of those infants whose patterns of movement are essentially normal but who exhibit slow or immature motor development. The AIMS should not, however, be used to follow motor development over time in infants who are diagnosed with a severe motor disorder involving abnormal patterns of movement.

Finally, the AIMS may be used to evaluate the motor development of infants who have no predisposing factors in their medical histories but who have been identified as having suspect development in routine medical examinations. These infants are typically full-term infants who have experienced no complications in the pre-, peri-, or neonatal periods. Physicians or public health nurses often identify these infants in well baby or immunization clinics. The AIMS may be used by these health professionals as an objective evaluation of the motor development of these infants, permitting the comparison of the infant's development to peers of the same age.

The AIMS should not be used to evaluate the motor abilities of older children whose motor skills are still at an infant level or to evaluate or monitor the motor development of infants with abnormal patterns of movement. Given the age limitations associated with the normative data for the AIMS, the interpretation of a score derived for a child older than 18 months would not be valid. It is also inappropriate to evaluate the motor abilities of older children on an infant scale of normal movement, even if their motor skills are at an infant level. Instead, their motor performance should be evaluated using a measure that assesses their functional level rather than their patterns of movement.

In the case of infants with abnormal patterns of movement, the abnormal components of their movement, such as spasticity, will prevent them from satisfying the minimum criteria required to pass items on the AIMS. As a result, their scores on the AIMS will remain unchanged even when their motor performance improves functionally. For example, an infant with spastic diplegia who has learned to pivot using the arms cannot pass the pivot item on the AIMS unless the arms and legs are used together. Since it is unlikely that the movement pattern in the lower extremities will ever meet the criteria to pass the pivot item, this infant cannot be credited for a new motor ability. This child would be more appropriately evaluated using a scale that has been specifically developed for children with motor disabilities. The AIMS is intended to evaluate the motor skills of infants with immature motor development but normal patterns of movement and to compare their scores on the AIMS with scores collected on a representative sample of age-matched, normally developing infants. Table 4–1 summarizes the appropriate use of the

TABLE 4–1
Appropriate Use of the AIMS

Identification of Motor Delays
All infants, 18 months or younger

Evaluation of Motor Development Over Time
All infants, 18 months or younger, except those with abnormal patterns of movement

AIMS in terms of infants who may be assessed according to the purpose of the assessment.

OBSERVATIONAL APPROACH

The AIMS has been intentionally designed as an observational assessment tool, thereby requiring minimal handling of an infant by the examiner. Although facilitation and handling are necessary elements of treatment, they should be consciously avoided when assessing an infant with the AIMS. Rather, the infant is encouraged to demonstrate the skills he or she can accomplish spontaneously, without the assistance of the examiner.

Pediatric physical and occupational therapists continually combine their observational and handling skills when they treat infants with disorders of movement. Therapists modify their intervention techniques in response to the reactions they observe in the infants, and handling is essential to obtain optimal responses from infants. Although competent handling is necessary for the effective treatment of infants with motor disorders, handling may be detrimental when introduced too soon or too extensively during the assessment of an infant's motor skills (Haley et al., 1986; Werner and Bayley, 1966).

Traditional testing of developmental markers such as primitive reflexes, muscle tone, and righting and equilibrium reactions often entails both extensive handling of an infant and the placement of the infant in arbitrary and stressful testing positions, such as vertical and horizontal suspension. This invasive style of testing can frighten and upset an infant, minimizing the possibility of observing an optimal response. In contrast, when a therapist observes an infant moving spontaneously, without touching or manipulating the child, the infant's integrated, functional movements can be observed and assessed, instead of the fragmented motor components of reflexes, reactions, and muscle tone.

A therapist's knowledge of motor development allows the identification of missing or deviant motor components without testing each unit separately. The lack of one age-appropriate reaction or reflex is not important if the infant is moving in a normal manner. Itemized, fragmented testing often results in a narrow analysis of movement skills. For example, a placing reaction that is lacking in a 6-month-old infant is insignificant if age-appropriate motor skills are present. Concern arises only when an infant's spontaneous movements are negatively affected by the presence of a cluster of abnormal components.

From the perspective of the dynamic motor theory, physical handling of an infant introduces a new environmental constraint into the context of the infant's movements. This new constraint can modify the spontaneous movements, making it difficult to observe and assess the infant's natural motor abilities. During the AIMS assessment, the infant, not the therapist, should initiate and execute the movements. The role of the therapist is to observe and analyze the infant's movements.

The observation of spontaneous movements also enables a therapist to identify the positive aspects of an infant's motor repertoire, providing a more balanced view of the infant's motor abilities. Traditional assessments of motor development have too often emphasized the documentation of the abnormal components of movement, such as the presence of an evoked asymmetrical tonic neck reflex or ankle clonus. A more challenging exercise than documenting the presence of an abnormal reflex is to observe an infant moving spontaneously and analyze how certain motor skills are accomplished in spite of the presence of an asymmetrical tonic neck reflex. Testing components of movement in isolation overemphasizes the negative findings; observing the infant move spontaneously permits the synthesis of both the positive and negative aspects of that movement.

The observational assessment approach also increases the social comfort level of the infant. Stranger anxiety is a normal stage of development for infants in the first year of life. Frequently, an infant becomes agitated and upset when handled by even a sensitive therapist, thus prohibiting further assessment. By using an observational assessment tool, a therapist may remain unobtrusive and distanced from the infant. Although the observational approach is often welcomed by parents and infants, therapists are sometimes uncomfortable merely observing an infant move, given their traditional focus on handling activities. For this reason, the ability to perform an observational assessment is often more difficult than eliciting a reflex or reaction through specific handling techniques.

EVALUATORS

The AIMS may be performed by any health professional who has a background in infant motor development and an understanding of the essential components of movement as described for each AIMS item. Evaluators must also have acquired skill in performing observational assessments of movement. Each evaluator should achieve an acceptable level of inter- and intra-rater reliability in administering the AIMS to a variety of infants prior to using the AIMS for clinical or research purposes.

TIME REQUIREMENTS

Twenty to 30 minutes is required to complete the entire assessment. A large portion of this time may be used for the infant to acclimate to the testing situation. Normally, once an infant begins moving, a series of items can be observed in a brief period. If the infant is upset or ill and a complete assessment cannot be obtained at one session, the remaining items may be readministered at any time up to 1 week after the original assessment.

MATERIALS NEEDED

Examining table for younger infants; (0 to 4 months)
Mat or carpeted area for older infants; the mat should be firm enough
    that it does not impede the infant's ability to move
Toys appropriate for ages 0 to 18 months
A stable wooden bench or chair to observe some of the pull to stand,
    standing, and cruising items in the standing subscale
AIMS score sheet and graph

SETTING

The assessment may be done in a clinic or in the home. A warm, quiet room is desirable. For the young infant, the assessment should be conducted on an examining table or other raised surface. After 4 months of age, infants should be examined on a mat or carpeted area. The usual precautions should be taken to ensure the safety of the infant during an assessment.

INFANT'S STATE

Whenever possible, the infant should be naked for the assessment. An infant who is anxious about removing clothes may be assessed wearing a diaper and shirt. After the infant has adapted to the assessment, the shirt may be removed to evaluate truncal posture.

The infant should be awake, active, and content during the assessment. The examiner and parent or parents may interact with the infant in any reasonable manner to achieve and maintain this optimal state. At times the examiner may have to distance himself or herself from the infant and observe from the corner of the room. If an infant continues to cry and cannot be comforted, the examination should be terminated and resumed at another date within 1 week of the interrupted assessment.

PARENT INVOLVEMENT

The parent or caregiver should be present during the assessment and should undress the infant. If the infant is anxious, the parent may comfort and position the infant for any items that require active placement or positioning.

PROMPTING

Certain items require positioning or physical prompting; these items are clearly specified in their descriptions. Otherwise, handling of the infant should be minimized. Visual and auditory prompts may be used by the examiner or parent as required. Toys may be employed to encourage or motivate the infant to move and explore the environment. The examiner may interact and play with the infant to encourage a response, but physical facilitation of a movement should be avoided.

If a specific prompt is required for an item, it is indicated in the item description. Younger infants who are not yet assuming the positions independently may be placed in the four different positions to assess their motor development. For example, an infant who does not yet assume the sitting position may be placed in this position to assess emerging sitting motor abilities. However, the examiner should not facilitate the motor abilities in any position.

SEQUENCING OF THE ASSESSMENT

It is not necessary to administer the entire scale to each infant. An infant should be tested only on those items in the range most appropriate for the infant's developmental level. Examiner discretion and parental reporting are used to determine the starting point on the scale for each infant.

Although the infant must be assessed in each of the four positions, the assessment does not have to follow any particular sequence. Nor does one item set have to be completed before observing the infant in another position. Items from the four subscales are observed as the infant moves naturally in and out of positions. If the infant is too young to move independently in and out of the four positions, the examiner or parent may place the infant in a position. Occasionally, an infant who is capable of moving from one position to another will not be motivated to do so during the course of the examination. For example, an infant aged 7 to 8 months of age is frequently happy in the prone position and will not spontaneously roll into the supine position even though the skill is in his or her repertoire. In order to observe movement in the supine position, it may be necessary for the parent or examiner to place the infant in this position.

SCORING

The score sheet consists of a line drawing for each item with key descriptors of postures or components of movements that *must* be observed in order for the infant to receive credit for the item. The examiner should consult Chapters 5 through 8 for a more complete description of the weight-bearing, posture, and antigravity movements associated with each item.

The scoring system entails a dichotomous choice for each item scored as either "observed" or "not observed"; no option exists for an infant to receive a score or partial credit for an item that is emerging. The examiner should complete the score sheet at the end of the assessment, not during the observational period. In this way, the examiner's attention is focused on observing and analyzing an infant's movements rather than on identifying each skill separately in order to complete the score sheet.

For each of the four positions, the least mature and most mature item observed during the assessment are identified and scored "observed." The items between the least and most mature "observed" items in each position represent the infant's possible motor repertoire in that position, his or her "window" of current skills. Each item within this window must then be scored either "observed" or "not observed"; *all* items within the window must be scored. An item is scored "observed" only if the examiner observed the item as depicted in the line drawing and described by the key descriptors on the score sheet during the assessment. No item may be credited on the basis of developmental assumptions or parental reporting. Occasionally, items within an infant's window may have already been mastered and discarded. However, if any items are within the window and are not observed during the assessment, for whatever reason, they must be scored "not observed." Figures 4–1 and 4–2 illustrate some possible scoring sequences.

Although there is no minimum or maximum number of trials for an infant to perform an item, the opportunity should be given for the infant to demonstrate the entire movement repertoire. For example, an infant who is just beginning to move spontaneously from a sitting to a prone position may initiate the movement many times before successfully completing it. If the examiner believes the infant is capable of completing the motor skill, he or she may be encouraged to attempt the movement a number of times. Sometimes it is necessary to leave an item and return to it later during the assessment. An assessment should not take longer than 30 minutes; if during this time an infant is happy and active and still has failed to perform a specific item, it is concluded that the item is not currently in the infant's motor repertoire.

In the scoring of bidirectional motor items such as rolling, pivoting, and cruising, the examiner should use clinical judgment. If after observing the infant move, the examiner has no concerns about symmetry, the infant may be credited for a bidirectional item even though it was observed in only one direction. In most instances an infant will move spontaneously in both directions. However, initially an infant may practice a new skill in only one direction; rolling from a supine to a prone position and pivoting are two examples of such skills. If the movement pattern is normal, and if the examiner has no concerns about symmetry, the item may be credited even though it has been observed in only one direction. If, however, the examiner doubts the infant's abilities to move symmetrically, the infant should be encouraged to perform the item in both directions. If, in this instance, the examiner is unable to motivate the infant to move in both directions and still retains a concern about asymmetry, the item should be scored "not observed."

To determine an infant's total AIMS score, the four positional scores—prone, supine, sitting, and standing—are calculated. Each item below the least mature item observed in each position is credited 1 point. Each "observed" item in the infant's motor window is credited 1 point. The sum of the credited points is the positional score. The sum of the four positional scores yields the infant's total score. See Tables 4–2 and 4–3 for scoring examples.

A summary of the scoring procedure follows.

To calculate a positional score:

Identify the least mature "observed" item in each position
Identify the most mature "observed" item in each position
The items between these two items are considered to be the infant's motor "window"
Score each item in the "window" as either "observed" or "not observed"
Credit 1 point to each item below the least mature "observed" item
Credit 1 point to each item scored "observed" within the infant's "window"
Sum the points to obtain a positional score
Sum the four positional scores to compute a total AIMS score

TABLE 4–2
Scoring: Sample Score Sheet 1

	Previous Items Credited	Items Credited in Window	Subscale Score
Prone	3	3	6
Supine	3	2	5
Sit	0	2	2
Stand	1	1	2
		Total Score 15	

Sample Score Sheet 1
O = "Observed"
NO = "Not Observed"

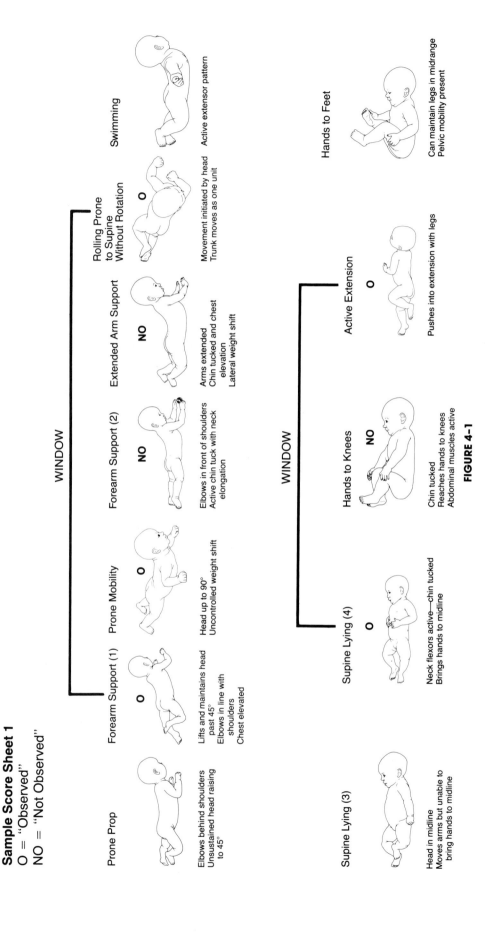

WINDOW

Prone Prop

Forearm Support (1)
O
Lifts and maintains head past 45°
Elbows in line with shoulders
Chest elevated

Prone Mobility
O
Head up to 90°
Uncontrolled weight shift

Forearm Support (2)
NO
Elbows in front of shoulders
Active chin tuck with neck elongation

Extended Arm Support
NO
Arms extended
Chin tucked and chest elevation
Lateral weight shift

Rolling Prone to Supine Without Rotation
O
Movement initiated by head
Trunk moves as one unit

Swimming
Active extensor pattern

Elbows behind shoulders
Unsustained head raising to 45°

WINDOW

Supine Lying (3)
Head in midline
Moves arms but unable to bring hands to midline

Supine Lying (4)
O
Neck flexors active—chin tucked
Brings hands to midline

Hands to Knees
NO
Chin tucked
Reaches hands to knees
Abdominal muscles active

Active Extension
O
Pushes into extension with legs

Hands to Feet
Can maintain legs in midrange
Pelvic mobility present

FIGURE 4-1

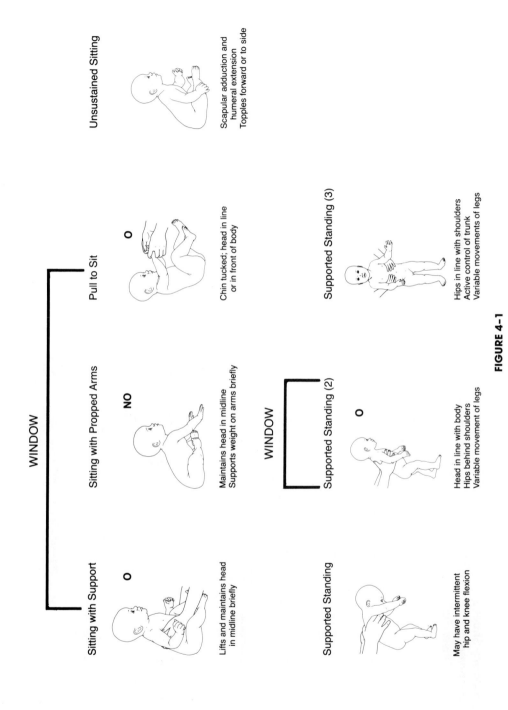

WINDOW

Sitting with Support

o

Lifts and maintains head
in midline briefly

Sitting with Propped Arms

NO

Maintains head in midline
Supports weight on arms briefly

Pull to Sit

o

Chin tucked; head in line
or in front of body

Unsustained Sitting

Scapular adduction and
humeral extension
Topples forward or to side

Supported Standing

May have intermittent
hip and knee flexion

WINDOW

Supported Standing (2)

o

Head in line with body
Hips behind shoulders
Variable movement of legs

Supported Standing (3)

Hips in line with shoulders
Active control of trunk
Variable movements of legs

FIGURE 4-1

Sample Score Sheet 2
O = "Observed"
NO = "Not Observed"

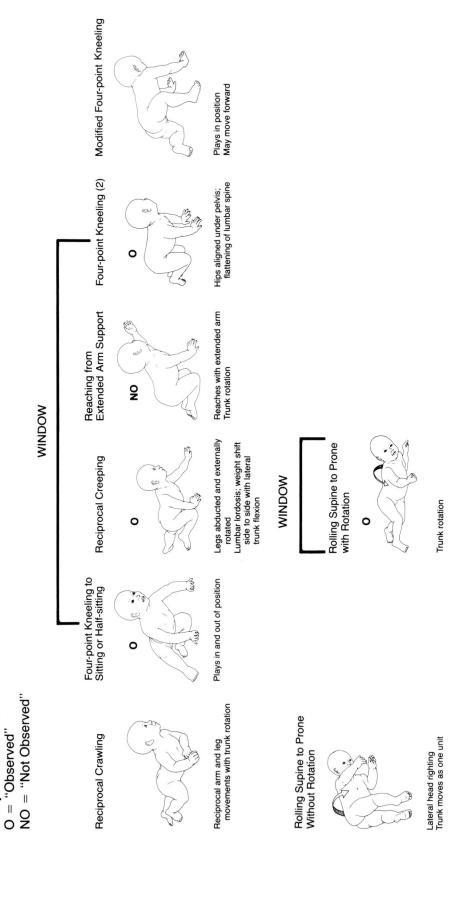

WINDOW

Four-point Kneeling to
Sitting or Half-sitting

O

Plays in and out of position

Reciprocal Creeping

O

Legs abducted and externally
rotated
Lumbar lordosis; weight shift
side to side with lateral
trunk flexion

Reaching from
Extended Arm Support

NO

Reaches with extended arm
Trunk rotation

Four-point Kneeling (2)

O

Hips aligned under pelvis;
flattening of lumbar spine

Modified Four-point Kneeling

Plays in position
May move forward

Reciprocal Crawling

Reciprocal arm and leg
movements with trunk rotation

WINDOW

Rolling Supine to Prone
with Rotation

O

Trunk rotation

Rolling Supine to Prone
Without Rotation

Lateral head righting
Trunk moves as one unit

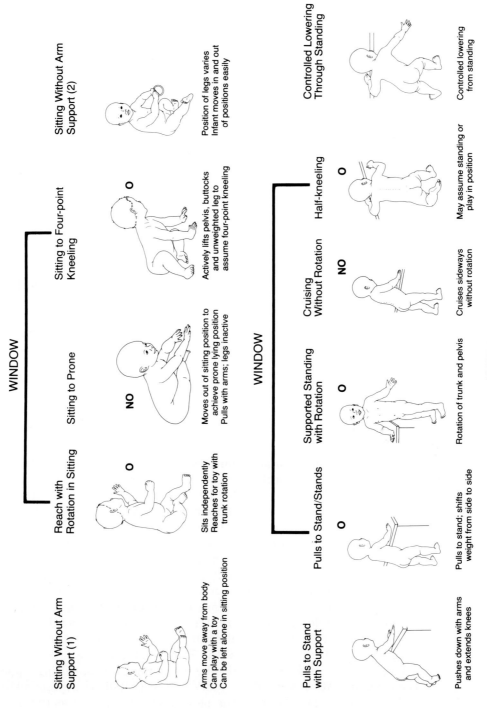

WINDOW

Sitting Without Arm Support (1)

Reach with Rotation in Sitting

Sitting to Prone

NO

Sitting to Four-point Kneeling

O

Sitting Without Arm Support (2)

Arms move away from body
Can play with a toy
Can be left alone in sitting position

Sits independently
Reaches for toy with trunk rotation

Moves out of sitting position to achieve prone lying position
Pulls with arms; legs inactive

Actively lifts pelvis, buttocks and unweighted leg to assume four-point kneeling

Position of legs varies
Infant moves in and out of positions easily

WINDOW

Pulls to Stand with Support

Pulls to Stand/Stands

O

Supported Standing with Rotation

O

Cruising Without Rotation

NO

Half-kneeling

O

Controlled Lowering Through Standing

Pushes down with arms and extends knees

Pulls to stand; shifts weight from side to side

Rotation of trunk and pelvis

Cruises sideways without rotation

May assume standing or play in position

Controlled lowering from standing

FIGURE 4-2

TABLE 4–3
Scoring: Sample Score Sheet 2

	Previous Items Credited	Items Credited in Window	Subscale Score
Prone	15	3	18
Supine	8	1	9
Sit	8	2	10
Stand	4	3	7
		Total Score 44	

PLOTTING THE SCORES

A graph is provided to plot the infant's total AIMS score (see Appendix I). From this graph, the examiner can determine the percentile ranking of the infant's motor performance compared with the normative age-matched sample of infants. To obtain an infant's percentile ranking, the infant's age, in months and weeks, is calculated using the following method:

EXAMPLE 1

	Year	Month	Day
Date of Assessment:	1993	12	10
Date of Birth:	1993	4	5
Age at Assessment:		8	5

EXAMPLE 2

	Year	Month	Day
		13	40
Date of Assessment:	~~1993~~	~~2~~	~~10~~
Date of Birth:	1992	9	30
Age at Assessment:		4	10

In Example 2, for calculation purposes each month contains 30 days and each year contains 12 months. For an infant born at less than 37 weeks gestation, corrected age is calculated by subtracting the days of prematurity from the age at assessment. Days of prematurity are calculated by subtracting the child's gestational age (in weeks) from 40 weeks (full-term).

The infant's age is located on the horizontal axis of the graph. The infant's total AIMS score is located on the vertical axis. A perpendicular line is drawn from each of these points; the percentile ranking of the infant's score may be determined from the point of intersection of these two lines. The information derived from plotting the child's score on the graph yields a single-point estimation of the child's percentile ranking. For example, if an infant who is 4 months, 1 week old receives a total AIMS score of 13, the percentile ranking on the graph would occur just below the 25th percentile.

The percentile ranking may also be determined by consulting Appendix II. The column that contains the infant's age is located. The infant's score is located in the raw score column. The percentile rank located at the intersection of the infant's raw score and the age group represents the percentile rank compared with the scores of infants in the same age grouping. Because the percentile ranks listed in Appendix II have been averaged over the entire age month, it is important to recognize that the listed percentiles are less accurate for infants whose ages fall at the extremes of the age grouping, such as an infant who is 4 months, 1 day old or an infant who is 4 months, 28 days old.

The percentile ranking indicates what proportion of the normative sample of infants of the same age obtained a similar score. For example, a 60th percentile ranking for a 4-month-old infant indicates that 60% of the infant's peers obtained a score equal to or less than that obtained by the assessed infant and that only 40% of similar infants obtained a higher score.

The higher the percentile ranking, the less likely that the infant is demonstrating a delay in motor development. For instance, an 80th or 90th percentile ranking clearly indicates that the infant's total score is equal to or greater than 80 or 90% of his or her peers, with only 10 or 20% of peers obtaining a higher score. The interpretation of a lower percentile is less clear. A 10th percentile ranking suggests that only 10% of the infant's peers obtained a lower score, thereby causing some reason for concern. Clearly, the lower the percentile ranking, the more likely the infant is to be exhibiting atypical motor development for age. Because the AIMS is not a diagnostic test and because the long-term predictive validity of the AIMS is not yet known, the specific implications of low percentile rankings are not definitive. The action to be taken as a result of a low percentile ranking, such as ongoing monitoring, referral for further diagnostic work-up, or intervention for motor delays, must be determined by the examiner in light of the child's performance and age, coupled with the examiner's clinical judgment.

References

Haley SM, Harris SR, Tada WL, et al.: Item reliability of the Movement Assessment of Infants. Phys Occup Ther Pediatr 1986; 6:21–39.

Lansford A: The high risk infant. In: Krajicek MJ, Tearney AI (eds): *Detection of Developmental Problems in Children.* Baltimore, University Park Press, 1977, pp 79–87.

Werner EE, Bayley N: The reliability of Bayley's revised scale of mental and motor development during the first year of life. Child Dev 1966; 37:39–50.

five

PRONE SUBSCALE

_____
_____
_____
_____
_____
_____
_____
_____
_____
_____
_____
_____
_____
_____
_____
_____
_____
_____
_____
_____
_____
_____
_____
_____
_____
_____
_____
_____
_____

The prone subscale contains 21 items. Each item consists of an artist's drawing of an infant accompanied by a photograph of a baby performing the movement. A detailed description of the weight bearing, posture, and antigravity movements observed in each position is included with each item. These descriptions are more detailed than the key descriptors provided on the score sheet. The examiner should refer to the more detailed descriptions of the item for clarification of the weight bearing, posture, and antigravity movements associated with each item. In order to receive credit for an item, the infant must exhibit all of the key descriptors noted on the score sheet.

The examiner may place a very young infant in the prone position. However, for older infants who are moving across the four subscales spontaneously, no physical handling is required to score the prone items.

Each item is accompanied by a graph depicting the percentage of infants in the normative sample for each age category that received credit for the particular item. On each graph, the *x*-axis indicates the age in months, and the *y*-axis represents the percentage of infants receiving credit for the item. A solid line has been drawn to indicate the age at which 50% of infants received credit for the item. A dotted line has been drawn at the age at which 90% of infants successfully completed the item. For example, in the *prone mobility* item, 50% of 3-month-old infants and 90% of 4-month-old infants successfully performed this item. These graphs provide information on the frequency distribution of the age of attainment of each skill.

Prone Lying (1)

Weight Bearing	Weight on cheek, hands, forearms, and upper chest
Posture	Head rotated to one side Physiological flexion Arms close to body; elbows flexed
Antigravity Movement	Turns head to clear nose from surface

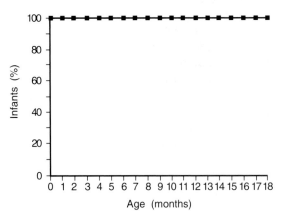

Prone lying (1)

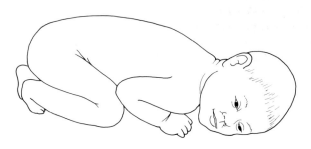

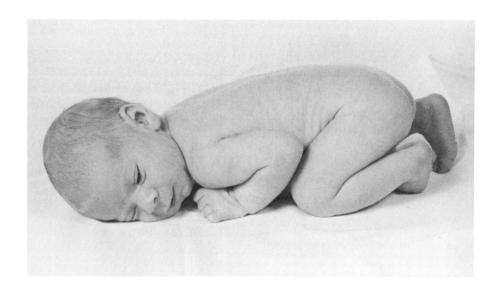

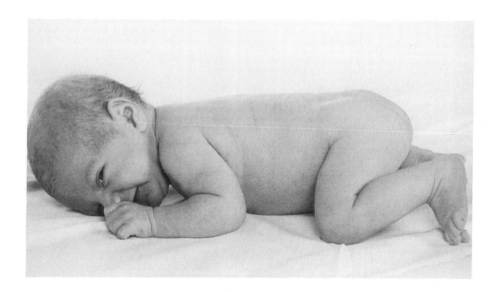

Prone Lying (2)

Weight Bearing	Weight on hands, forearms, and chest
Posture	Elbows behind shoulders and close to body Hips and knees flexed
Antigravity Movement	Lifts head asymmetrically to 45° Cannot maintain head in midline

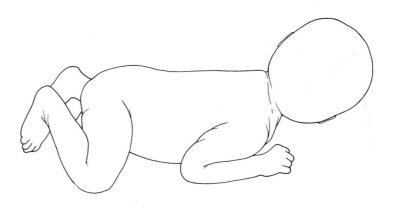

Prone lying (2)

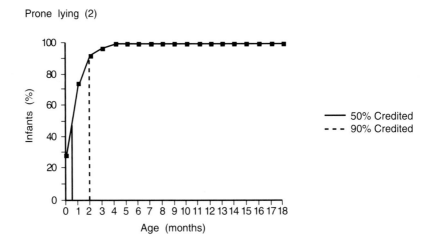

— 50% Credited
- - - 90% Credited

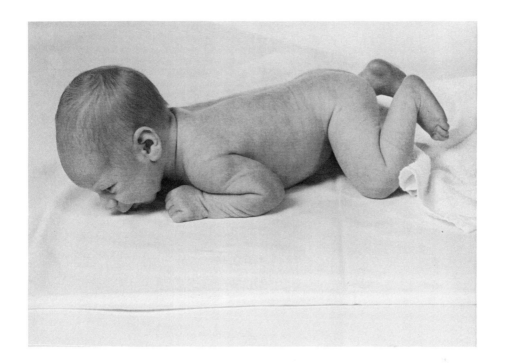

Prone Prop

Weight Bearing	Weight on hands, forearms, and chest
Posture	Shoulders slightly abducted Elbows behind shoulders Hip and knees flexed
Antigravity Movement	Raises head to 45° Turns head

The infant is able to lift the head to 45° in the midline; this position may not be maintained indefinitely.

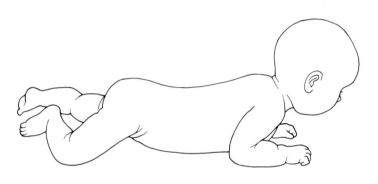

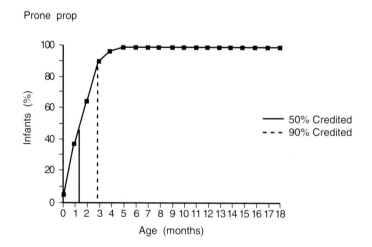

Prone prop

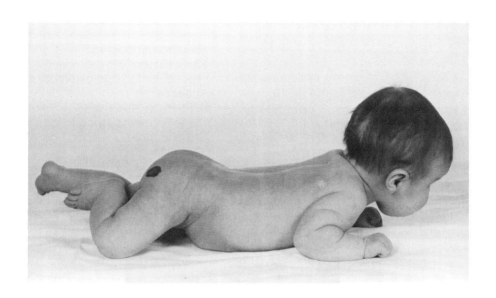

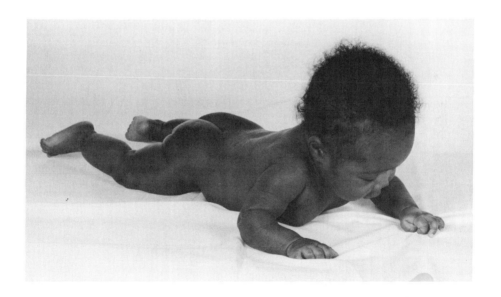

Forearm Support (1)

Weight Bearing	Weight symmetrically distributed on forearms and trunk
Posture	Shoulders abducted Elbows in line with shoulders Hips abducted and externally rotated Knees flexed
Antigravity Movement	Pushes against surface to raise head Lifts and maintains head past 45° Chest elevated

To pass this item the elbows must not be behind the shoulders; they may be beyond the shoulders. The infant may play with the feet together in this position. The head does not have to be maintained at 90°. Active chin tuck is not present.

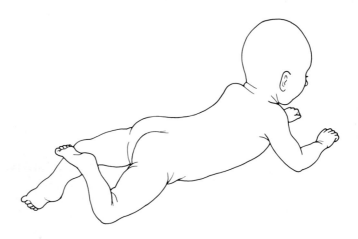

Forearm support (1)

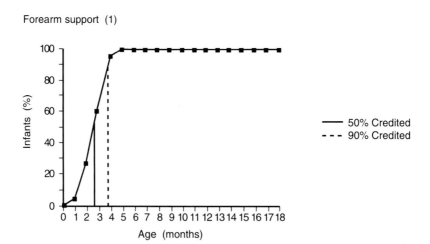

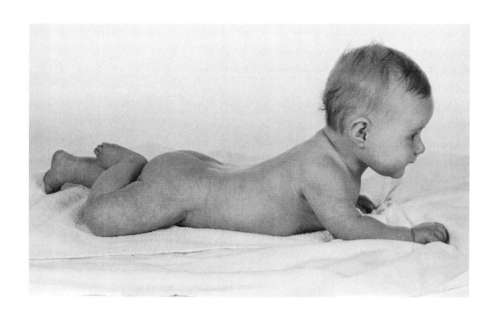

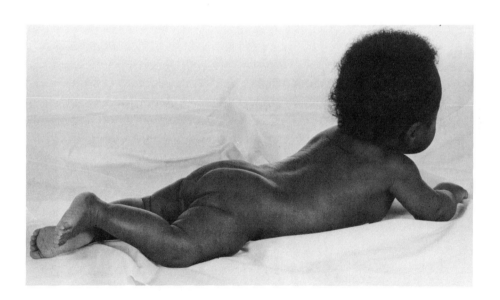

Prone Mobility

Weight Bearing	Weight on forearms, abdomen, and thighs
Posture	Head to 90° Forearm support or immature extended arm support Hips abducted
Antigravity Movement	Uncontrolled weight shift onto one arm; there may or may not be any displacement of the trunk

This item represents the infant's early attempts at weight shift in prone position.

Prompt: May place toys appropriately to observe antigravity movements.

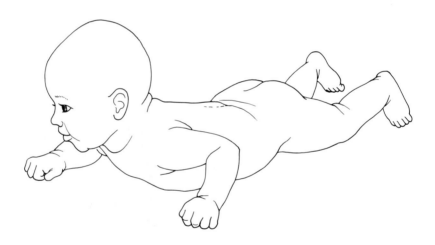

Prone mobility

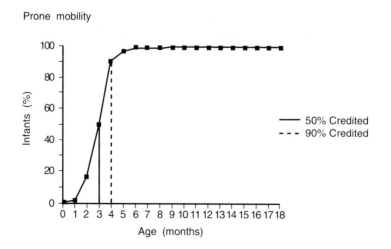

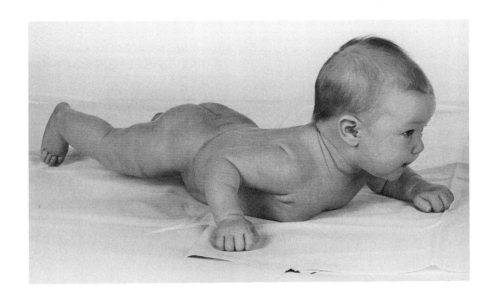

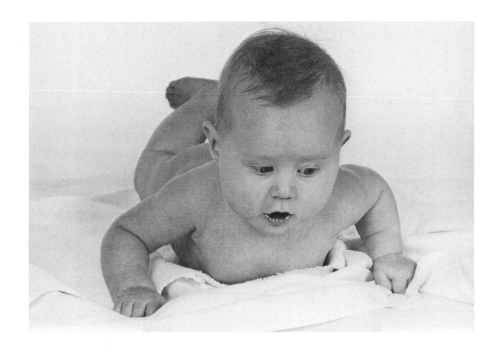

Forearm Support (2)

Weight Bearing	Weight on forearms, hands, and abdomen
Posture	Elbows in front of shoulders Hips abducted and externally rotated
Antigravity Movement	Raises and maintains head in midline Active chin tuck and neck elongation Chest elevated

The elbows must be in front of the shoulders to pass this item. The shoulders may be either abducted or in a more neutral position. The infant will often actively flex and extend the knees in this position. This item represents more mature head control than does the previous forearm support.

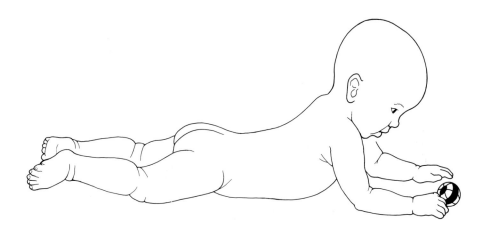

Forearm support (2)

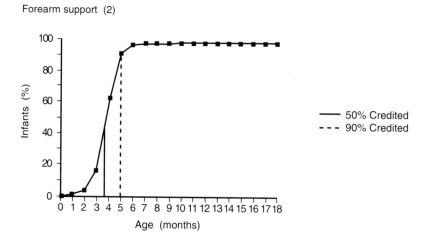

—— 50% Credited
- - - 90% Credited

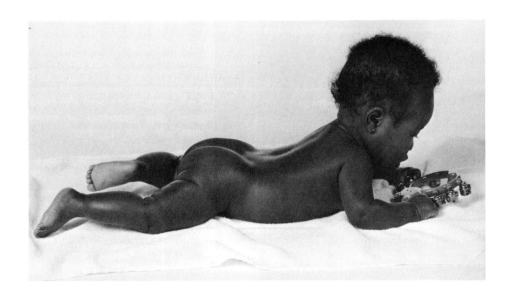

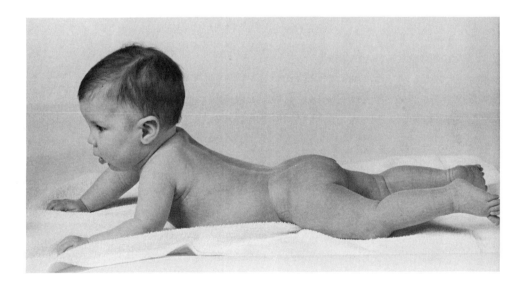

Extended Arm Support

Weight Bearing	Weight on hands, lower abdomen, and thighs
Posture	Arms extended Elbows in front of shoulders Legs approaching neutral position
Antigravity Movement	Chin tucked and chest elevated Flexion and extension of knees; may play with feet together Lateral weight shift

The infant may also push backward in this position.

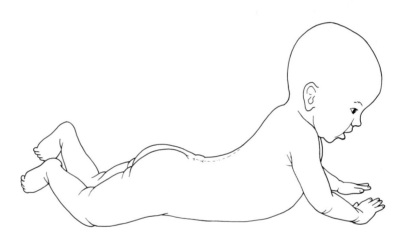

Extended arm support

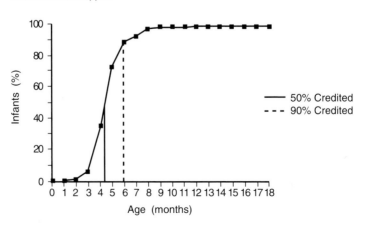

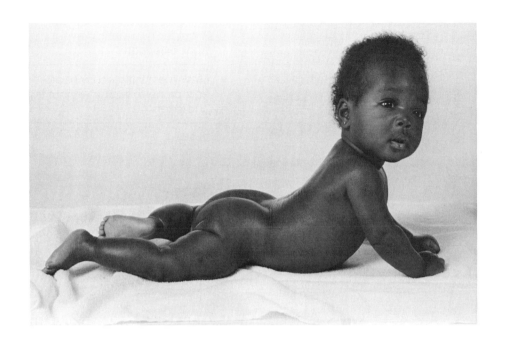

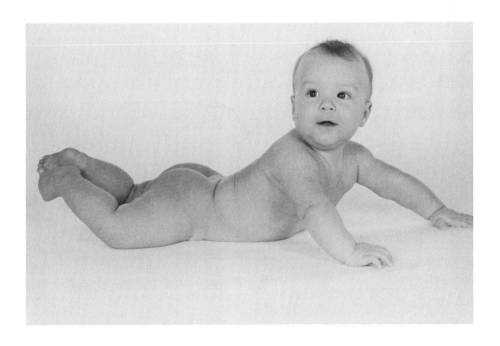

Rolling Prone to Supine Without Rotation

Weight Bearing	Weight on one side of body
Posture	Shoulder in line with pelvis Trunk extension
Antigravity Movement	Movement initiated by head Rolls prone to supine without trunk rotation

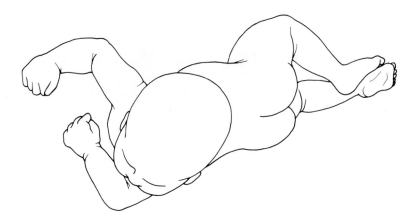

Rolling prone to supine without rotation

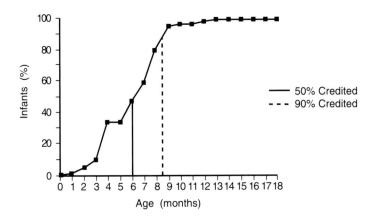

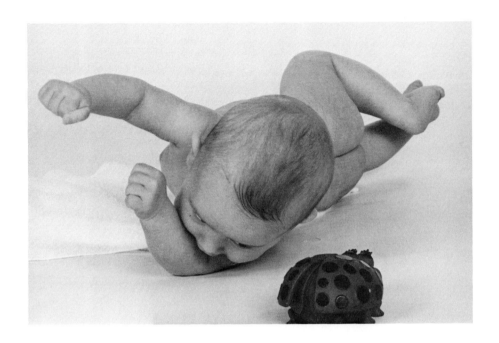

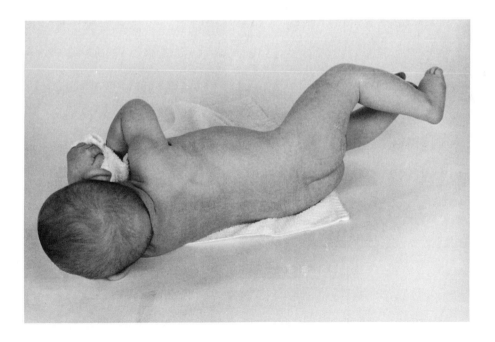

Swimming

Weight Bearing	Weight on abdomen
Posture	Symmetrical Scapulae adducted Arms abducted, externally rotated Legs abducted and extended Lumbar spine extended
Antigravity Movement	Raises head and arms or legs, or both, from surface Active extensor pattern

The infant may rock forward, backward, or side to side. There is no forward motion of the body and sometimes the extensor activity is seen only in the arms or the legs. There should always be some active extension observed in the trunk.

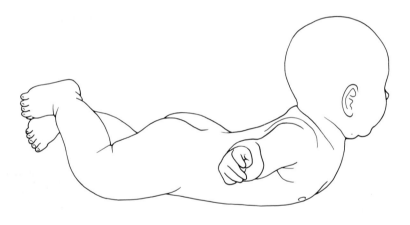

Swimming

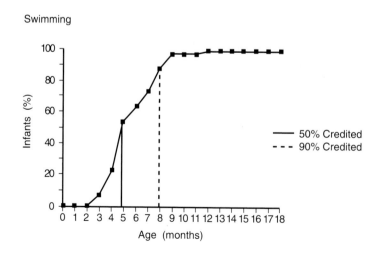

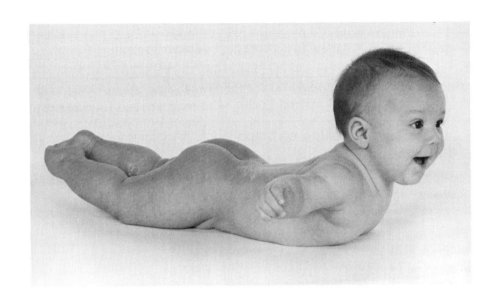

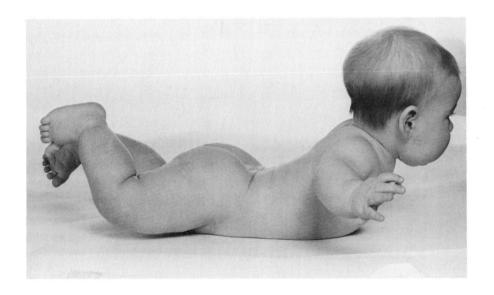

Reaching from Forearm Support

Weight Bearing	Weight on one forearm, hand, and abdomen
Posture	Forearm support Legs approaching neutral position
Antigravity Movement	Active weight shift to one side Controlled reach with free arm

This item represents a controlled reach; the infant does not lose his or her balance as the arm reaches.

Prompt: Object placed in midline or laterally to observe antigravity movements.

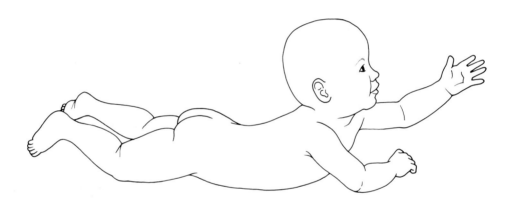

Reaching from forearm support

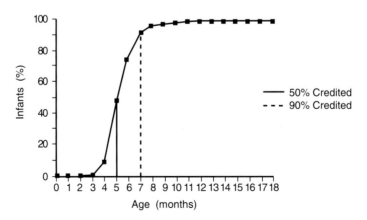

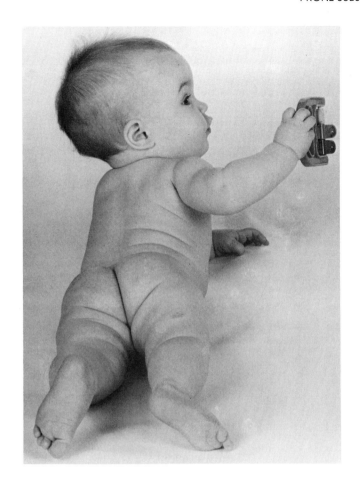

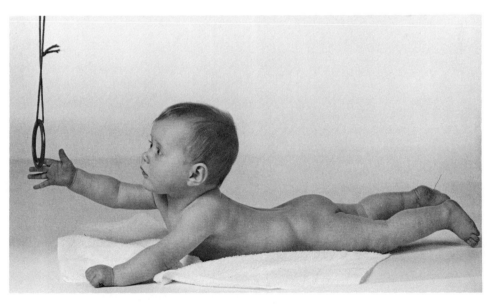

Pivoting

Weight Bearing	Weight on trunk, arms, and hands
Posture	Head to 90° Legs abducted and externally rotated
Antigravity Movement	Pivots Movement in arms and legs Lateral trunk flexion

To pass this item, the infant must use both arms and legs to pivot.

Prompt: Place toy laterally to initiate movement.

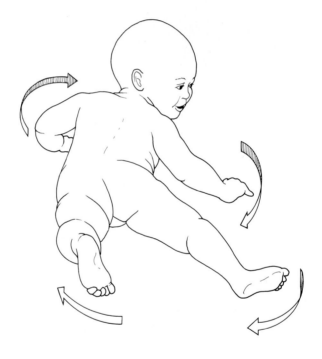

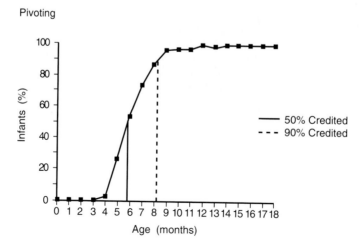

Pivoting

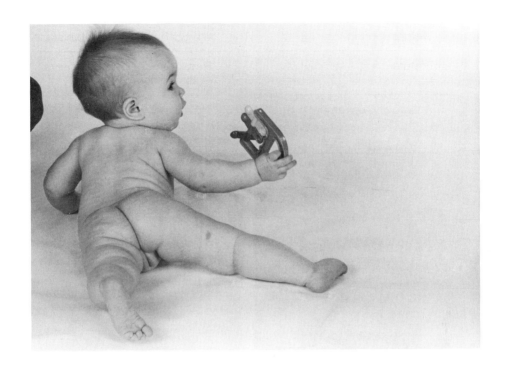

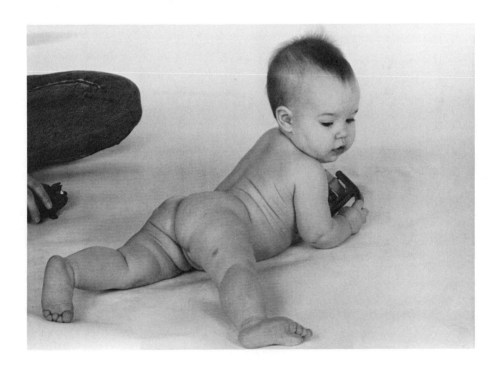

Rolling Prone to Supine with Rotation

Weight Bearing	Weight on one side of body
Posture	Shoulder not in line with pelvis Trunk rotation
Antigravity Movement	Movement initiated by shoulder, pelvis, or head Trunk rotation

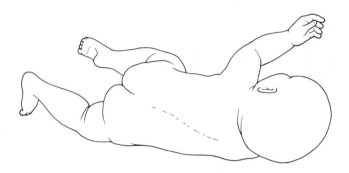

Rolling prone to supine with rotation

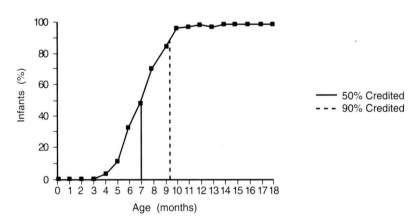

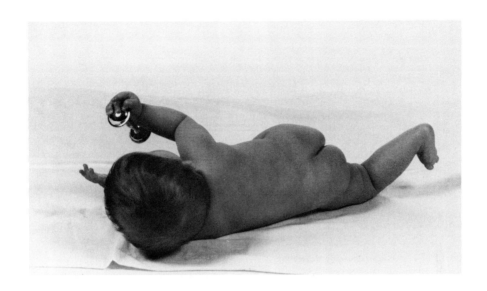

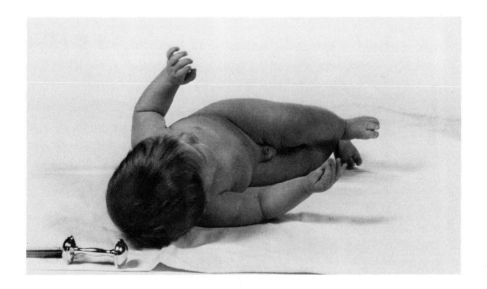

Four-Point Kneeling (1)

Weight Bearing	Weight on hands and knees
Posture	Legs flexed, abducted, and externally rotated Lumbar lordosis
Antigravity Movement	Maintains position May rock back and forth or diagonally May propel self forward by falling

This item is characterized by the immature posture of hip abduction. The shoulders may be internally rotated or in a neutral position. The infant need not be observed rocking to pass this item.

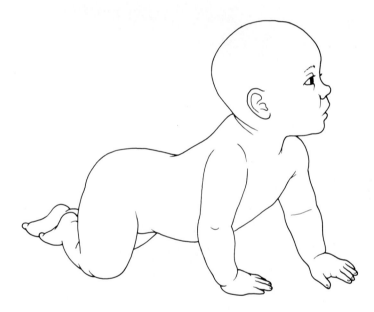

Four-point kneeling (1)

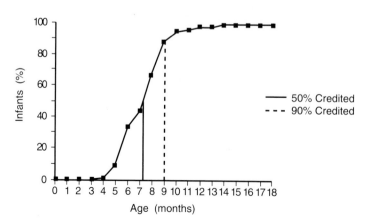

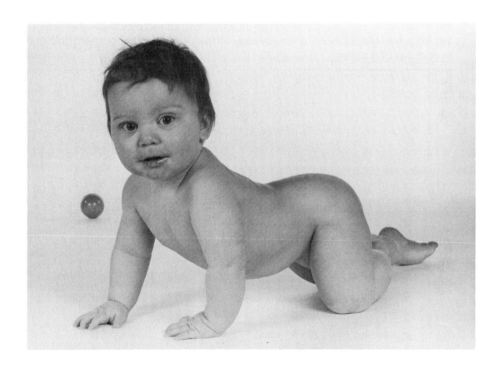

Propped Lying on Side

Weight Bearing	Weight on elbow, forearm, leg, and one side of trunk
Posture	Lateral head righting Lateral trunk flexion Upper leg flexed and adducted or abducted
Antigravity Movement	Dissociation of legs Shoulder stability Uses upper arm for reaching Rotation within body axis

The posture of the upper leg may change from hip abduction to adduction; the important features are shoulder stability and at least partial dissociation of one leg from the other. The infant may stay in this position only momentarily and move in and out of it often.

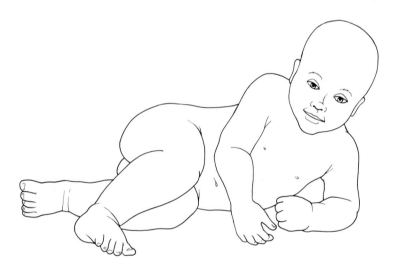

Propped on side

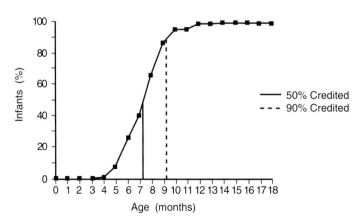

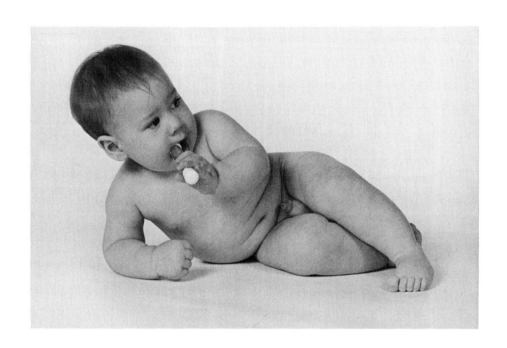

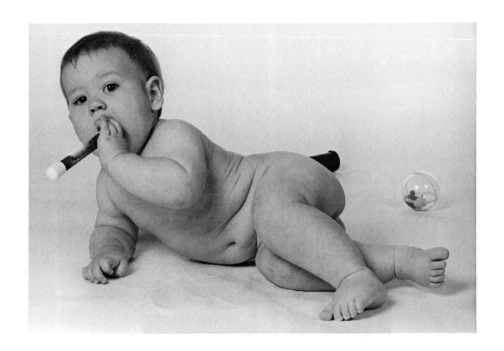

Reciprocal Crawling

Weight Bearing	Weight on opposite arm and leg
Posture	Flexion of one hip, extension of the other Arm flexion Head to 90° Rotation in trunk
Antigravity Movement	Reciprocal arm and leg movements with trunk rotation

Movement in both arms and legs must be observed.

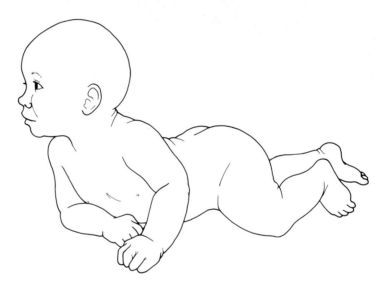

Reciprocal crawling

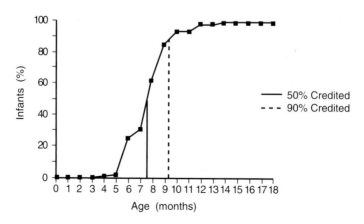

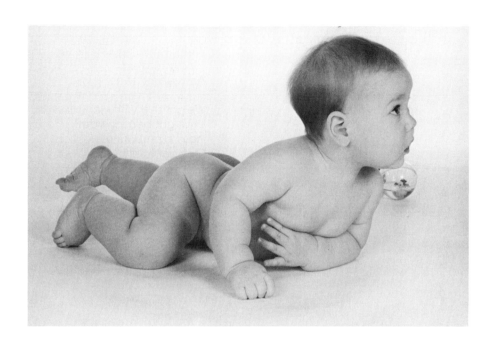

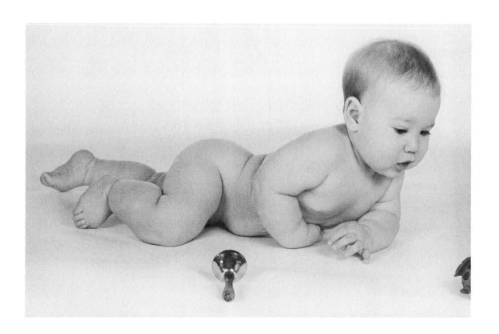

Four-Point Kneeling to Sitting or Half-Sitting

Weight Bearing	Weight on hands, leg, and foot on one side of body and other foot
Posture	Weight-bearing leg flexed and externally rotated Arms abducted
Antigravity Movement	Weight shift with elongation of trunk on weight-bearing side Plays in and out of position May get to sitting

The infant does not have to achieve sitting to pass this item; the midposition may follow four-point kneeling. Controlled movement of the pelvis is present.

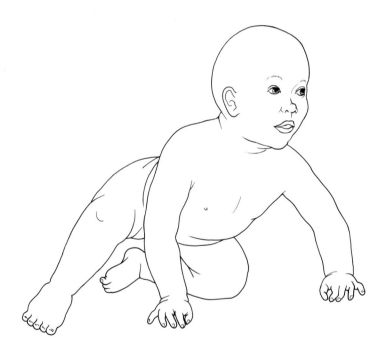

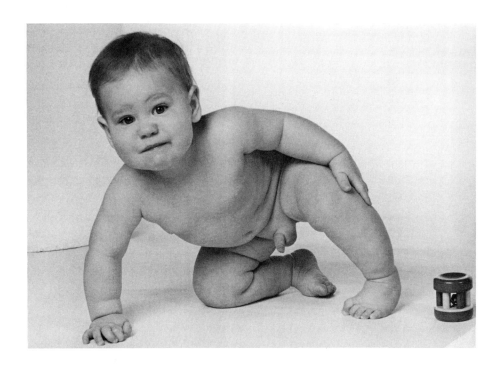

Four-point kneeling to sitting or half-sitting

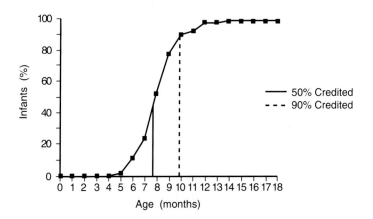

Reciprocal Creeping (1)

Weight Bearing	Weight on opposite hand and knee
Posture	Arms abducted Legs abducted and externally rotated Lumbar lordosis
Antigravity Movement	Weight shift side to side with lateral trunk flexion Reciprocal arm and leg movements

This is an early creeping pattern characterized by the immature posture of the legs and lack of trunk rotation. The infant must move forward to pass this item.

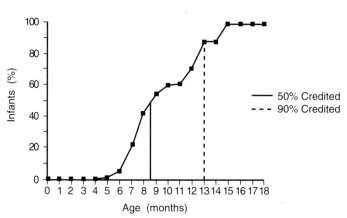

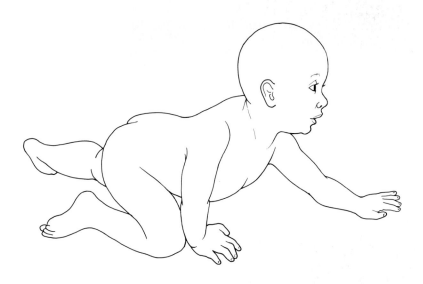

Reciprocal creeping (1)

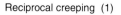

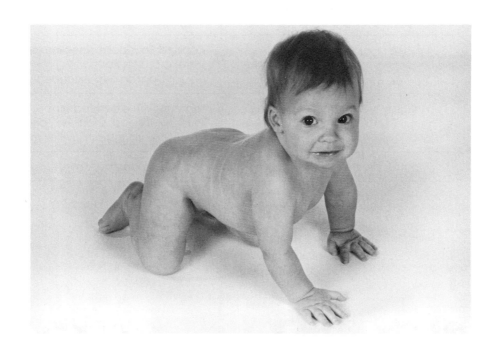

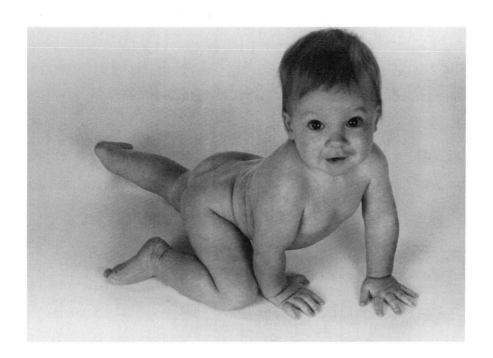

Reaching from Extended Arm Support

Weight Bearing	Weight on knees and one hand
Posture	Modified four-point kneeling with one arm off surface Weight-bearing arm extended
Antigravity Movement	Reaches with extended arm Rotation of head, shoulders, and trunk Weight-bearing arm may flex minimally

Prompt: May place toys appropriately to observe antigravity movements.

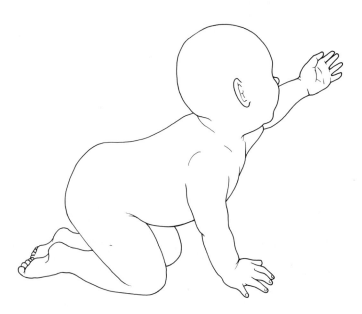

Reaching from extended arm support

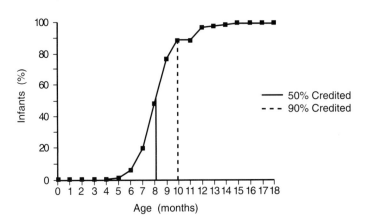

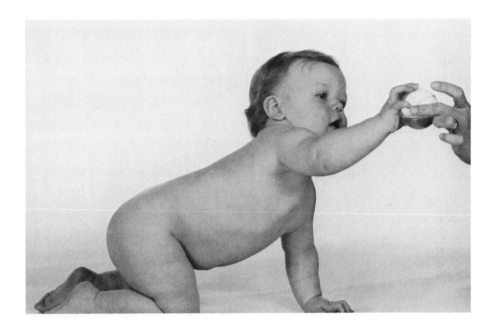

Four-Point Kneeling (2)

Weight Bearing	Weight on hands and knees
Posture	Legs flexed, hips aligned under pelvis Flattening of lumbar spine
Antigravity Movement	Abdominal muscles active Rocks back and forth and diagonally May propel self forward

This item is characterized by the mature posture of the hips aligned under the pelvis. The infant should either rock or creep forward to pass this item.

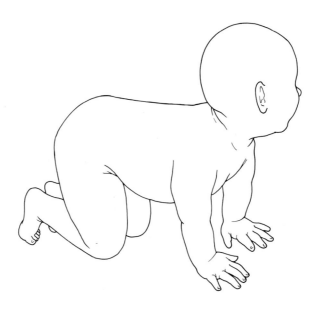

Four-point kneeling (2)

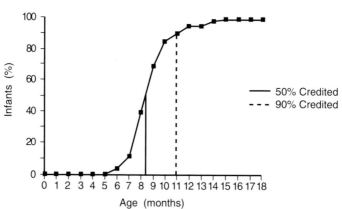

— 50% Credited
- - - 90% Credited

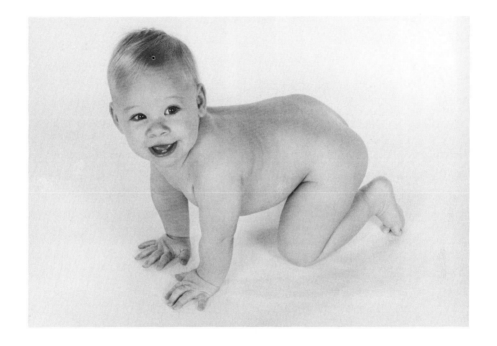

Modified Four-Point Kneeling

Weight Bearing	Weight on hands, one knee, and opposite foot
Posture	Modified quadruped position; one leg flexed at hip so that foot is plantigrade
Antigravity Movement	Plays in position May move forward

The flexed hip may be aligned under the pelvis or externally rotated. This is not a transitional movement to independent standing. It represents a variation of the four-point kneeling position.

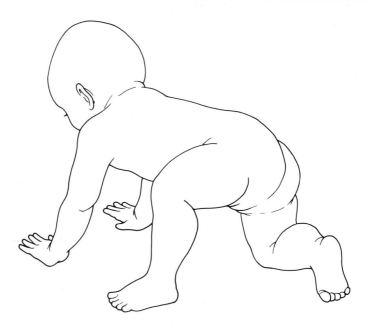

Modified four-point kneeling

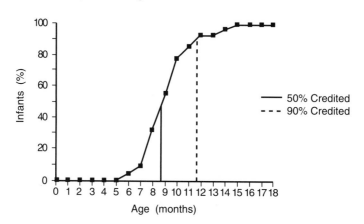

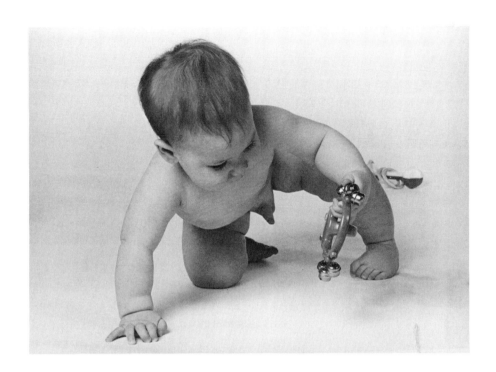

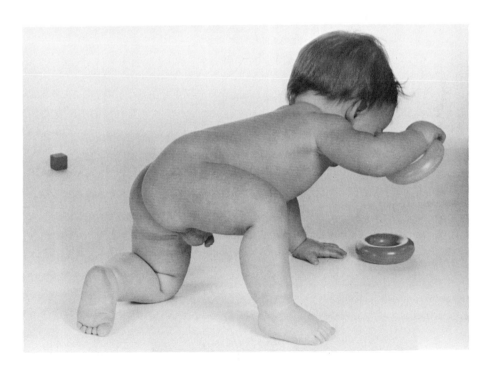

Reciprocal Creeping (2)

Weight Bearing	Weight on opposite hand and knee
Posture	Elbows and knees aligned under shoulders and hips Lumbar spine flat
Antigravity Movement	Reciprocal arm and leg movements with trunk rotation

This is a mature creeping pattern characterized by the mature posture of the legs and trunk rotation. Lumbar lordosis is not present.

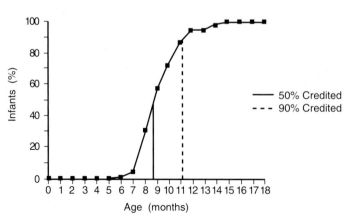

Reciprocal creeping (2)

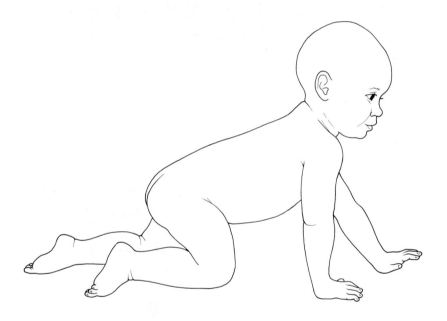

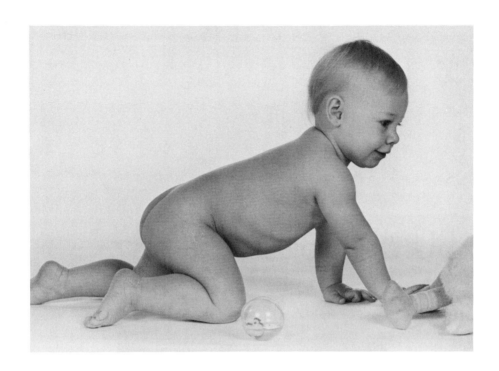

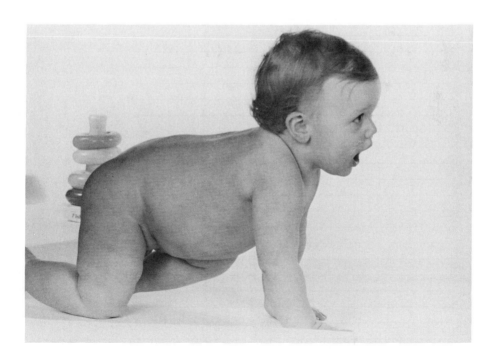

six

SUPINE SUBSCALE

_____
_____
_____
_____
_____
_____
_____
_____
_____
_____
_____
_____
_____
_____
_____
_____
_____
_____
_____
_____
_____
_____
_____
_____
_____
_____
_____

The supine subscale contains nine items. Each item consists of an artist's drawing of an infant accompanied by a photograph of a baby performing the movement. A detailed description of the weight bearing, posture, and antigravity movements observed in each position is included with each item. These descriptions are more detailed than the key descriptors provided on the score sheet. The examiner should refer to the more detailed descriptions of the item for clarification of the weight bearing, posture, and antigravity movements associated with each item. In order to receive credit for an item, the infant must exhibit all of the key descriptors noted on the score sheet.

The examiner may place a very young infant in the supine position. The supine subscale has the least number of items because as infants mature they do not stay in the supine position for long periods. Rather, they prefer to play in prone, sitting, or standing positions. As a result, the supine items are often not observed in an older infant. The examiner may ask the parent or caregiver to place an infant in the supine position in order to observe the pattern of rolling, but it is not expected that a series of supine items will be observed spontaneously in an older infant.

Each item is accompanied by a graph depicting the percentage of infants in the normative sample for each age category that received credit for the particular item. On each graph, the x-axis indicates the age in months, and the y-axis represents the percentage of infants receiving credit for the item. A solid line has been drawn to indicate the age at which 50% of infants received credit for the item. A dotted line has been drawn at the age at which 90% of infants successfully completed the item. For example, in the *hands to feet* item, 50% of 4.5-month-old infants and 90% of 6-month-old infants successfully performed this item. These graphs provide information on the frequency distribution of the age of attainment of each skill.

Supine Lying (1)

Weight Bearing	Weight on face, side of head, and trunk
Posture	Head rotated to one side Physiological flexion
Antigravity Movement	Head rotation Mouth to hand Random arm and leg movements (stretching)

The infant may move out of the flexed posture but returns to flexion as the resting posture.

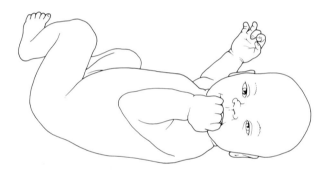

Supine lying (1)

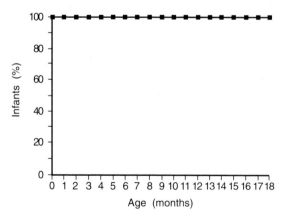

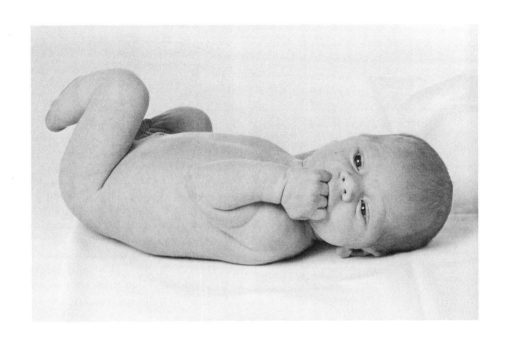

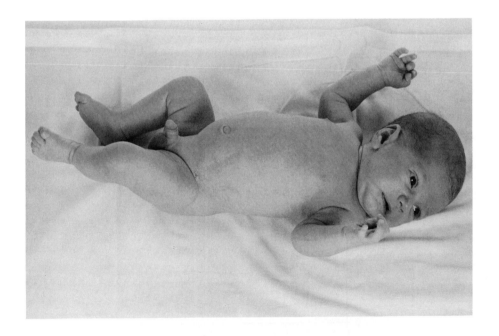

Supine Lying (2)

Weight Bearing	Weight on side of head, trunk, and buttocks
Posture	Physiological flexion diminishing Head rotated to one side Hips abducted and externally rotated Hands open or closed
Antigravity Movement	Head rotation toward midline Random arm and leg movements Nonobligatory asymmetrical tonic neck reflex may be present

The infant may move the head toward midline but cannot maintain the midline position.

Prompt: May use visual stimulus for head rotation.

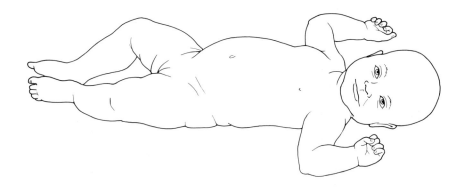

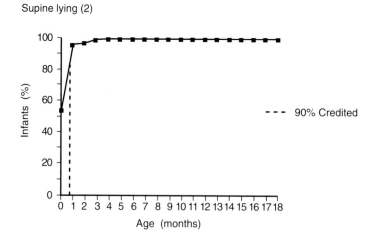

Supine lying (2)

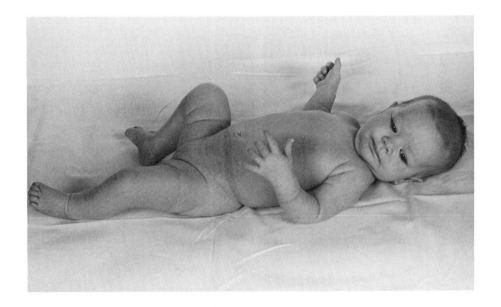

Supine Lying (3)

Weight Bearing	Weight symmetrically distributed on head, trunk, and buttocks
Posture	Head in midline Arms flexed and abducted or positioned at side of body Legs flexed or extended
Antigravity Movement	Bilateral or reciprocal kicking Moves arms but unable to bring hands to midline

The posture of the legs may vary between flexion and extension. The infant is still moving the arms at the side rather than playing in midline.

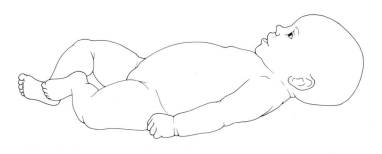

Supine lying (3)

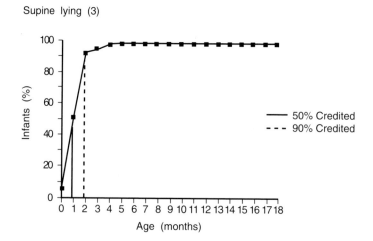

— 50% Credited
--- 90% Credited

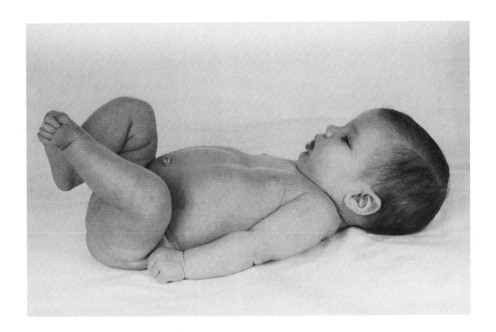

Supine Lying (4)

Weight Bearing	Weight symmetrically distributed on head, trunk, and buttocks
Posture	Head in midline with chin tuck Arms resting on chest Legs flexed or extended
Antigravity Movement	Neck flexors active—chin tuck Brings hands to midline Bilateral or reciprocal kicking

The infant is easily able to bring the hands together in the midline but does not have to successfully grasp a toy to pass this item.

Prompt: May use toy to observe progression of hands to midline.

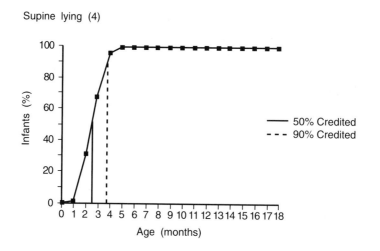

Supine lying (4)

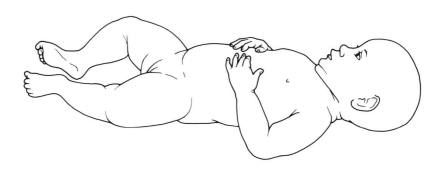

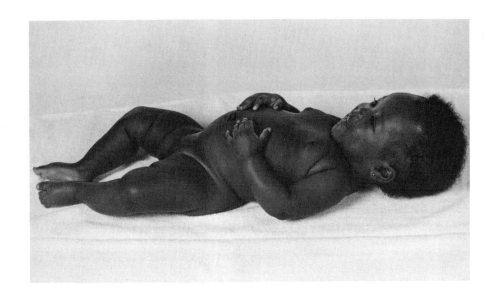

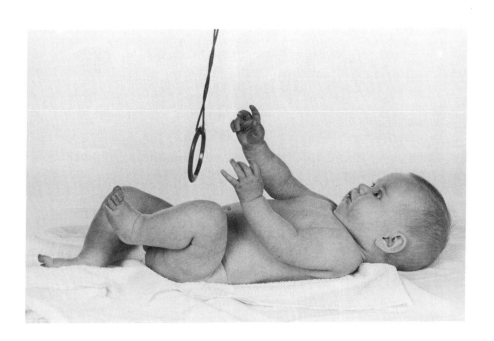

Hands to Knees

Weight Bearing	Weight symmetrically distributed on head, trunk, and pelvis
Posture	Hips abducted and externally rotated Knees flexed
Antigravity Movement	Turns head easily side to side Chin tuck Reaches hand or hands to knees Abdominal muscles active May fall to side by lifting legs

It is important to observe active abdominal muscles. If the legs are widely abducted and resting on the abdomen passively, the infant will not pass this item. Hypotonic infants often display this passive position.

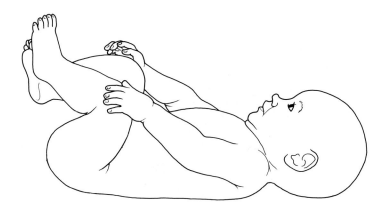

Hands to knees

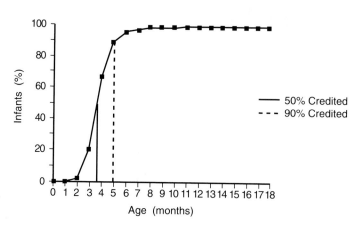

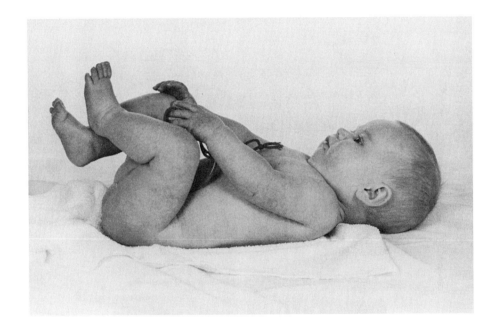

Active Extension

Weight Bearing	Weight on one side of body
Posture	Hyperextension of neck and spine
Antigravity Movement	Shoulders protracted Pushes into extension with one or both legs May roll to side accidentally

During this movement, one buttock usually remains on the supporting surface. This is a movement that the infant plays with, distinguishing it from the "arching" of hypertonic infants.

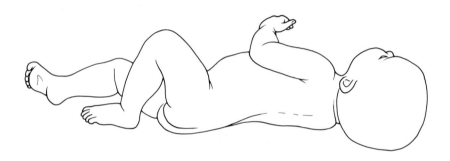

Active extension

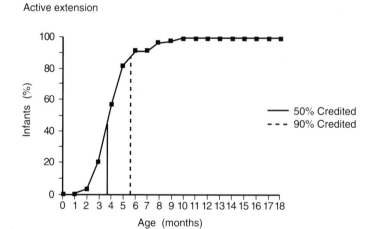

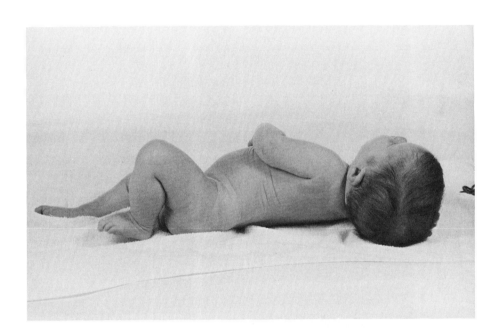

Hands to Feet

Weight Bearing	Weight on head and trunk
Posture	Hand contact with one or both feet Hips flexed greater than 90° Knees semiflexed or extended
Antigravity Movement	Chin tuck Lifts legs and brings feet to hands Can maintain legs in midrange Pelvic mobility present Rocks from side to side; may roll to side

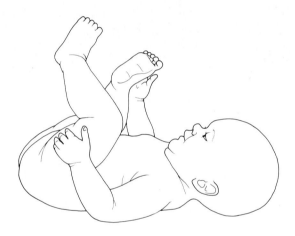

Hands to feet

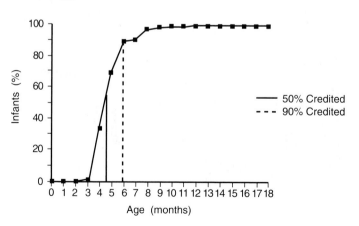

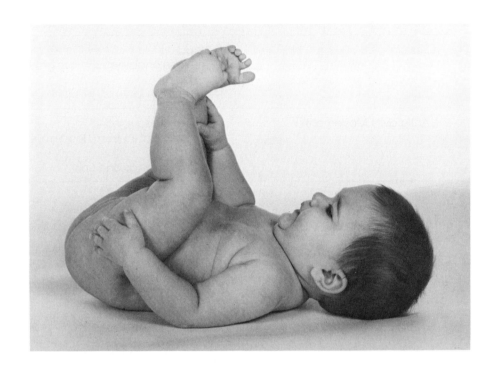

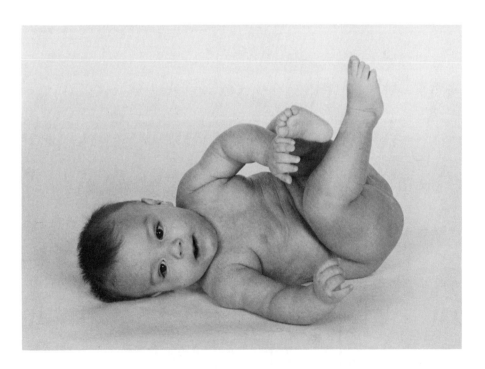

Rolling Supine to Prone Without Rotation

Weight Bearing	Weight on one side of body
Posture	Head up Trunk elongated on weight-bearing side Shoulder in line with pelvis
Antigravity Movement	Lateral head righting Rolling initiated from head, shoulder, or hip Trunk moves as one unit

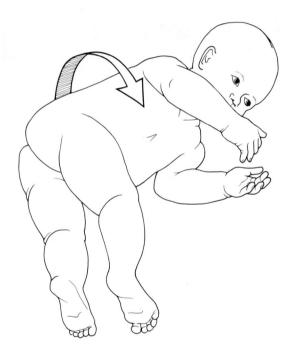

Rolling supine to prone without rotation

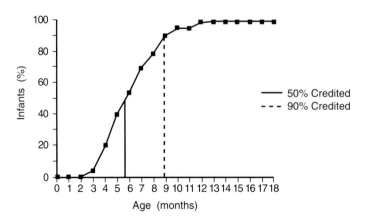

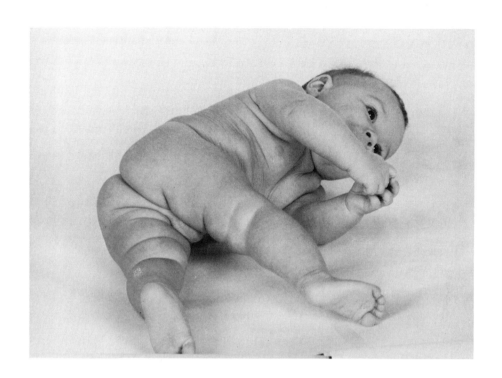

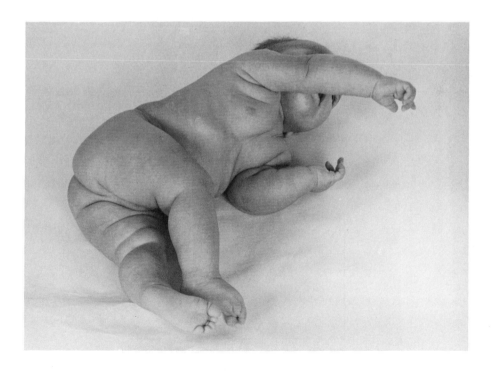

Rolling Supine to Prone with Rotation

Weight Bearing	Weight on one side of body
Posture	Head up Trunk elongated on weight-bearing side Shoulder and pelvis not aligned
Antigravity Movement	Lateral head righting Dissociated movement in legs Rolling initiated from head, shoulder, or hip Trunk rotation

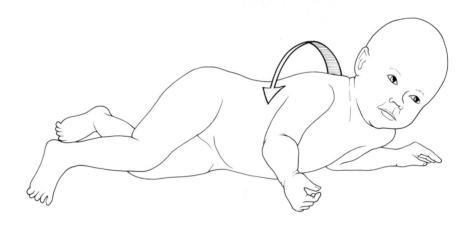

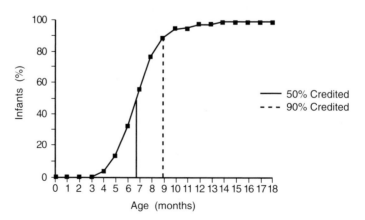

Rolling supine to prone with rotation

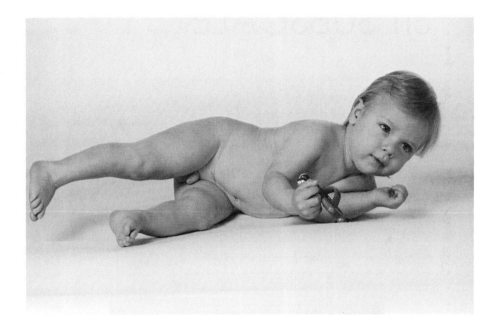

seven

SIT SUBSCALE

_____
_____
_____
_____
_____
_____
_____
_____
_____
_____
_____
_____
_____
_____
_____
_____
_____
_____
_____
_____
_____
_____
_____
_____
_____
_____

The sit subscale contains 12 items. Each item consists of an artist's drawing of an infant accompanied by a photograph of a baby performing the movement. A detailed description of the weight bearing, posture, and antigravity movements observed in each position is included with each item. These descriptions are more detailed than the key descriptors provided on the score sheet. The examiner should refer to the more detailed descriptions of the item for clarification of the weight bearing, posture, and antigravity movements associated with each item. In order to receive credit for an item, the infant must exhibit all of the key descriptors noted on the score sheet.

The first item, *sitting with support,* and the third item, *pull to sit,* require physical handling; all other items are observed without assistance from the examiner. Since an infant usually maintains sitting independently before being able to get in and out of the position independently, the examiner can place an infant in the sitting position in order to observe posture and movements.

Each item is accompanied by a graph depicting the percentage of infants in the normative sample for each age category that received credit for the particular item. On each graph, the *x*-axis indicates the age in months, and the *y*-axis represents the percentage of infants receiving credit for the item. A solid line has been drawn to indicate the age at which 50% of infants received credit for the item. A dotted line has been drawn at the age at which 90% of infants successfully completed the item. For example, in the *unsustained sitting* item, 50% of 4.5-month-old infants and 90% of 6-month-old infants successfully performed this item. These graphs provide information on the frequency distribution of the age of attainment of each skill.

Sitting with Support

Weight Bearing	Weight on buttocks and legs
Posture	Hip flexion Trunk flexion
Antigravity Movement	Lifts and maintains head in midline briefly Upper cervical spine extension

To pass this item, the infant must maintain the head in midline briefly. There must be more head control than "bobbing," but the head does not have to be maintained in midline indefinitely.

Prompt: The infant is supported by examiner around upper trunk.

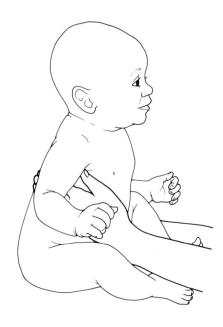

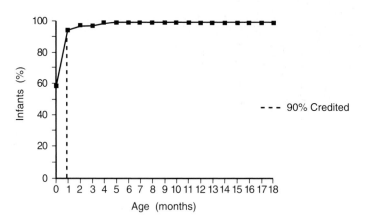

Sitting with support

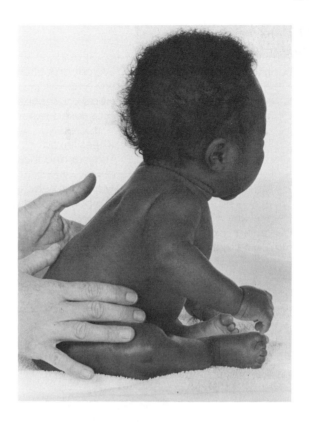

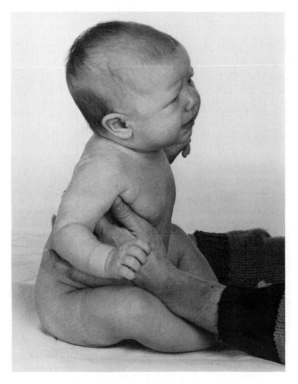

Sitting with Propped Arms

Weight Bearing	Weight on buttocks, legs, and hands
Posture	Head up; shoulders elevated Hips flexed, externally rotated, and abducted Knees flexed Lumbar and thoracic spine rounded
Antigravity Movement	Maintains head in midline Supports weight on arms briefly

Prompt: Examiner places the infant in sitting position. To pass this item, the infant must maintain the position independently without the examiner's support.

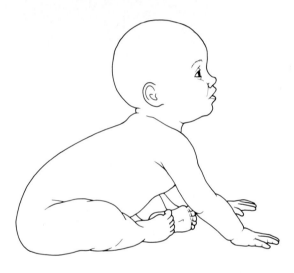

Sitting with propped arms

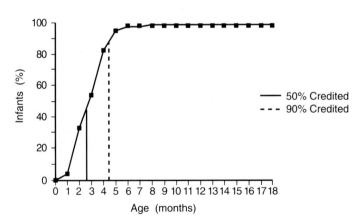

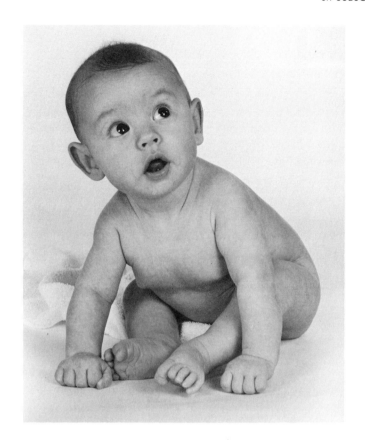

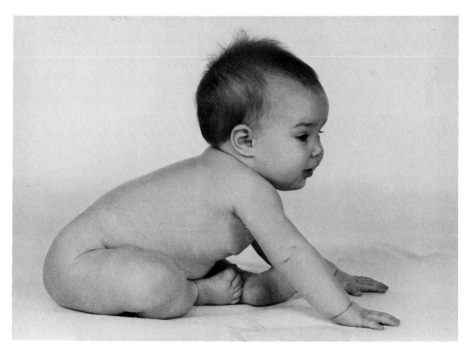

Pull to Sit

Weight Bearing	Weight on buttocks and lumbar spine
Posture	Arms flexed Hips and knees flexed Feet may be off surface
Antigravity Movement	Chin tucked; head in line or in front of body May assist movement with abdominal muscles and arm flexion

At the initiation of the movement, there may be a slight head lag, which the infant quickly overcomes. There may be varying degrees of flexion in the legs as the infant assists with the movement.

Prompt: Examiner pulls infant to sit by holding the wrists.

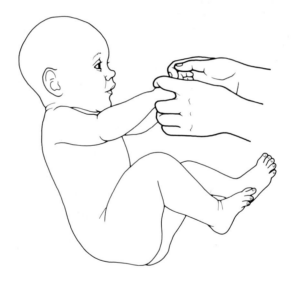

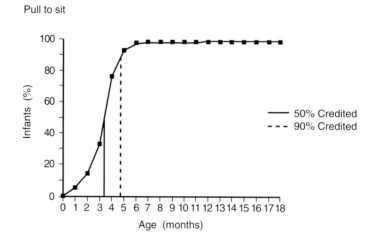

Pull to sit

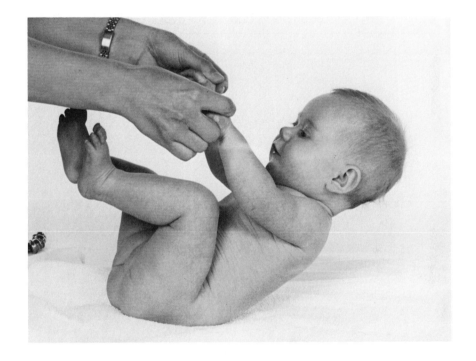

Unsustained Sitting

Weight Bearing	Weight on buttocks and legs
Posture	Head in midline Shoulders in front of hips Thoracic spine extended Lumbar flexion Hips flexed and externally rotated
Antigravity Movement	Head extension Scapular adduction and humeral extension Cannot maintain position indefinitely

Prompt: Examiner places infant in sitting position. To pass this item, the infant must maintain the position briefly and not fall over immediately.

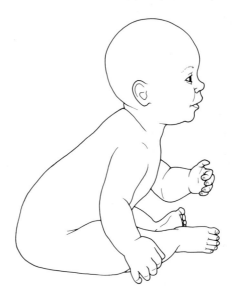

Unsustained sitting

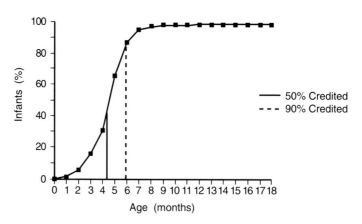

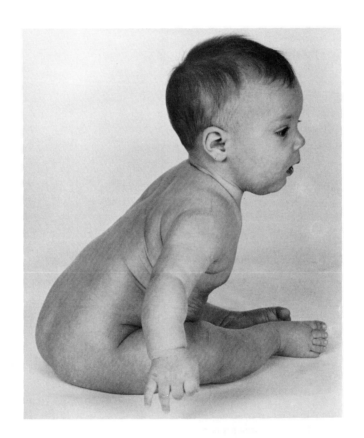

Sitting with Arm Support

Weight Bearing	Weight on buttocks, legs, and hands
Posture	Head up Lumbar spine rounded, thoracic spine extended Extended arm support Hips flexed, externally rotated, and abducted Knees flexed
Antigravity Movement	Head movements free from trunk Propped on extended arms Cannot move in and out of position

Prompt: Examiner places the infant in sitting position.

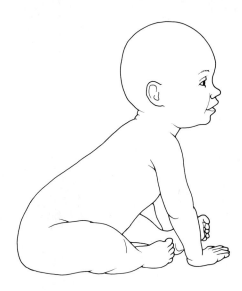

Sitting with arm support

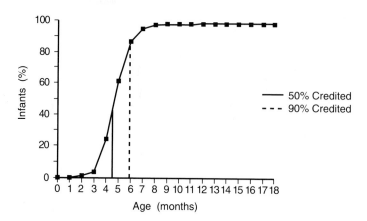

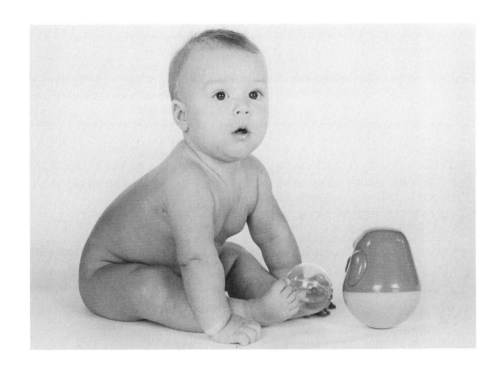

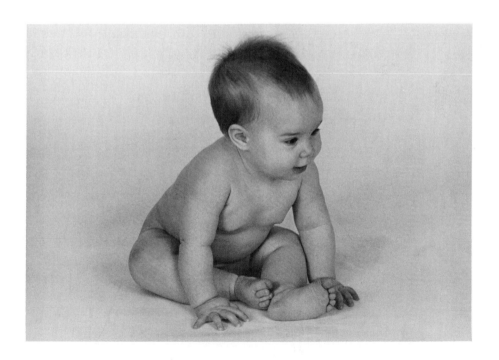

Unsustained Sitting Without Arm Support

Weight Bearing	Weight on buttocks and legs
Posture	Elbows flexed Thoracic spine extended Hips flexed, externally rotated, and abducted with wide base of support Knees flexed
Antigravity Movement	Cannot be left alone in sitting position indefinitely

To pass this item, the infant must be able to maintain sitting alone for a brief period but still may require supervision.

Prompt: Examiner places the infant in sitting position.

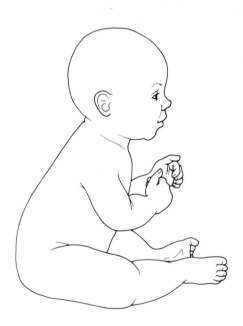

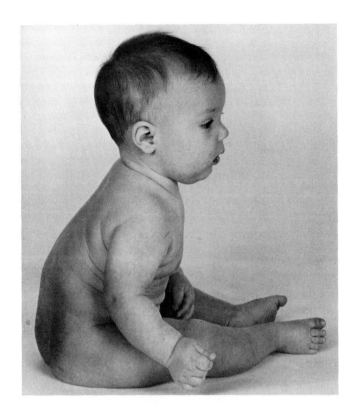

Unsustained sitting without arm support

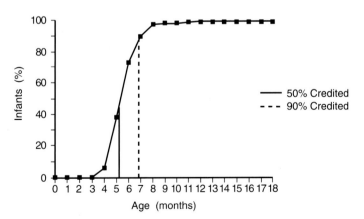

Weight Shift in Unsustained Sitting

Weight Bearing	Weight on buttocks and legs
Posture	Hips flexed, abducted, and externally rotated Arms free
Antigravity Movement	Weight shift forward, backward, or sideways Beginning to right body back to midline Cannot be left alone in sitting position

This item represents a stage in sitting in which an infant loses balance easily, especially when experimenting with weight shift.

Prompt: Examiner places the infant in sitting position. May use toys to elicit weight shift.

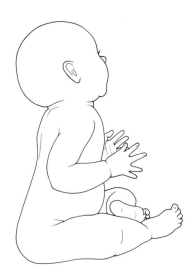

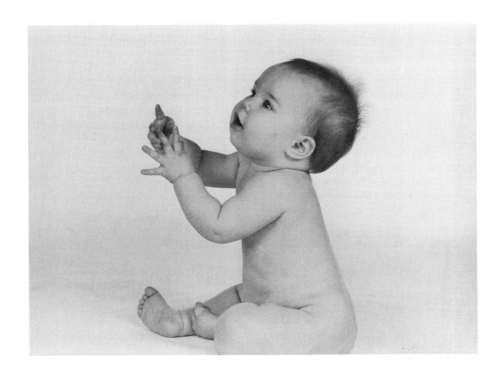

Weight shift in unsustained sitting

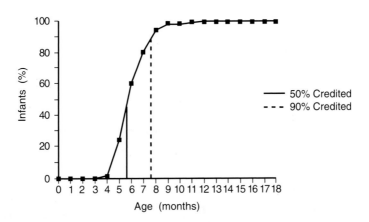

Sitting Without Arm Support (1)

Weight Bearing	Weight on buttocks and legs
Posture	Shoulders aligned over hips Arms free Wide base of support
Antigravity Movement	Arms move away from body Can play with a toy Can be left alone in sitting position

To pass this item, an infant must be able to maintain sitting well. The caregiver is comfortable leaving the infant in sitting position. Rotation within the trunk does not need to be present to pass this item.

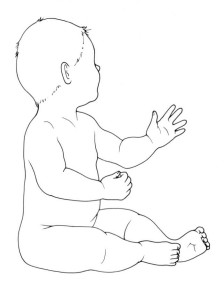

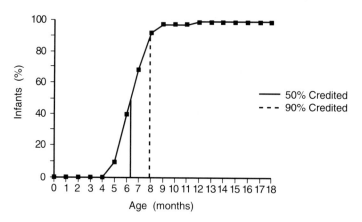

Sitting without arm support (1)

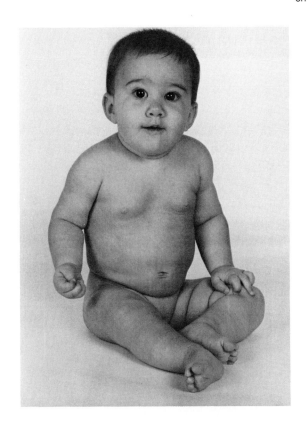

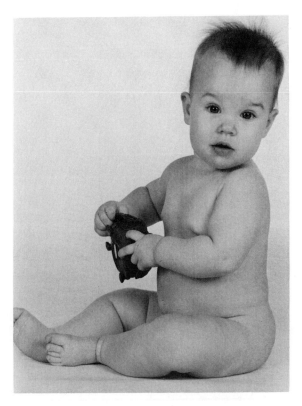

Reach with Rotation in Sitting

Weight Bearing	Weight on buttocks and legs
Posture	Trunk rotated Elongation of trunk on reaching side
Antigravity Movement	Sits independently Reaches for toy with trunk rotation

To pass this item, an infant must be able to easily reach for a toy, and rotation must be seen within the trunk. The infant may reach in any direction as long as trunk rotation is observed.

Prompt: Examiner may place infant in sitting position. May use toys to encourage infant to reach.

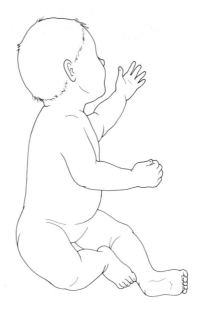

Reach with rotation in sitting

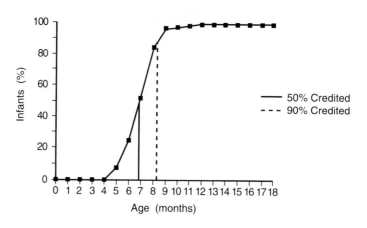

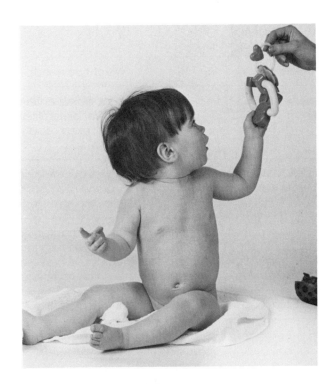

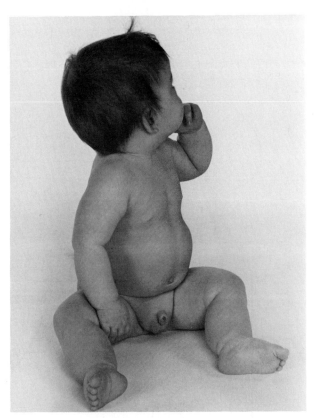

Sitting to Prone

Weight Bearing	Weight on hands, forearms, and trunk
Posture	Trunk flexed anteriorly or sideways over lower extremities Legs flexed, abducted, and externally rotated
Antigravity Movement	Moves out of sitting position to achieve prone lying position Pulls with arms; legs inactive

To pass this item, the infant must be able to maintain sitting with or without arm support. The infant may or may not use trunk rotation to get to prone position. This item is often observed as the infant's first attempt to move out of sitting position. The item can be passed even if it is performed in an immature manner.

Prompt: Examiner may place the infant in sitting position.

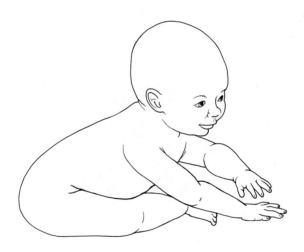

Sitting to prone

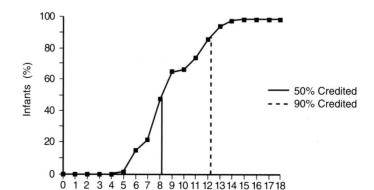

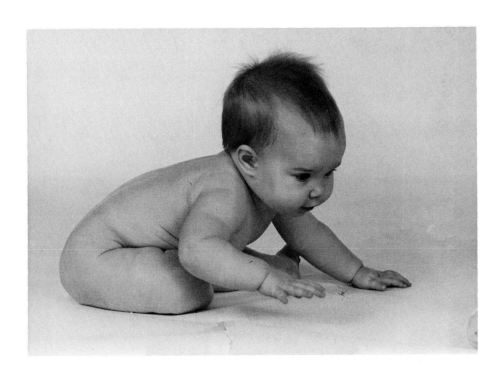

Sitting to Four-Point Kneeling

Weight Bearing	Weight on both hands and one foot
Posture	Moves from an independent sitting position to four-point kneeling
Antigravity Movement	Actively lifts pelvis, buttocks, and unweighted leg to assume four-point kneeling position

To pass this item the infant must be able to maintain sitting without arm support. A variety of ways may be demonstrated to assume four-point kneeling; the critical element is that it is a controlled movement and the pelvis is elevated—the infant cannot ''flop'' into prone position.

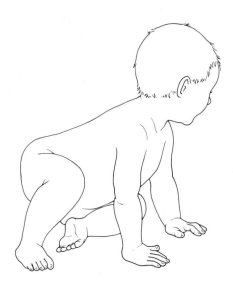

Sitting to four-point kneeling

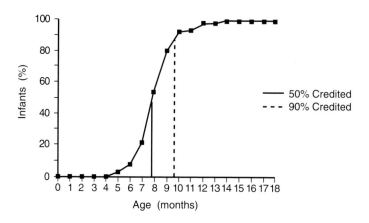

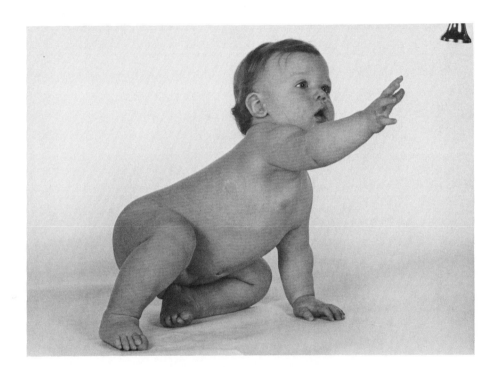

Sitting Without Arm Support (2)

Weight Bearing	Weight on buttocks
Posture	Variety of postures with dissociation of legs Narrow base of support
Antigravity Movement	Position of legs varies Infant moves in and out of positions easily

This item can be passed if a variety of sitting postures are observed; these include "W" sitting and side sitting. It is important to ascertain that the infant has more than one sitting posture in the movement repertoire. The infant must assume the position independently.

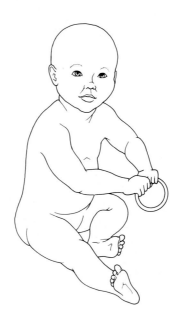

Sitting without arm support (2)

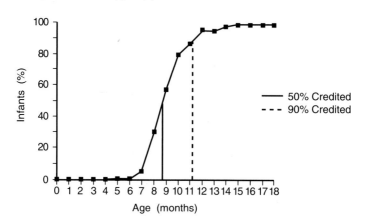

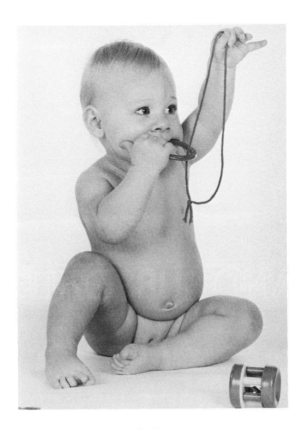

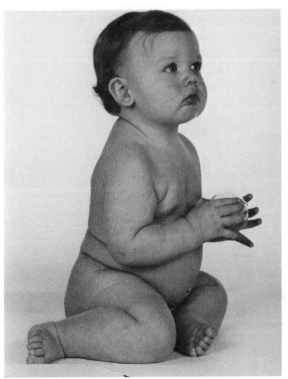

STAND SUBSCALE

_____
_____
_____
_____
_____
_____
_____
_____
_____
_____
_____
_____
_____
_____
_____
_____
_____
_____
_____
_____
_____
_____
_____
_____
_____
_____
_____

The stand subscale contains 16 items. Each item consists of an artist's drawing of an infant accompanied by a photograph of a baby performing the movement. A detailed description of the weight bearing, posture, and antigravity movements observed in each position is included with each item. These descriptions are more detailed than the key descriptors provided on the score sheet. The examiner should refer to the more detailed descriptors of the item for clarification of the weight bearing, posture, and antigravity movements associated with each item. In order to receive credit for an item, the infant must exhibit all of the key descriptors noted on the score sheet.

In order to observe the first three standing items, the examiner must support the infant in a standing position. To receive credit for any of the remaining items in the stand subscale the infant must assume standing independently.

Each item is accompanied by a graph depicting the percentage of infants in the normative sample for each age category that received credit for the particular item. On each graph, the x-axis indicates the age in months, and the y-axis represents the percentage of infants receiving credit for the item. A solid line has been drawn to indicate the age at which 50% of infants received credit for the item. A dotted line has been drawn at the age at which 90% of infants successfully completed the item. For example, in the *stands alone* item, 50% of 10.5-month-old infants and 90% of 13-month-old infants successfully performed this item. These graphs provide information on the frequency distribution of the age of attainment of each skill.

Supported Standing (1)

Weight Bearing	Bears weight intermittently
Posture	Head flexed forward Hips behind shoulders Hips and knees flexed Feet may be close together Infant does not slip through examiner's hands
Antigravity Movement	There may be intermittent hip and knee flexion

Prompt: Supported by examiner under axillae.

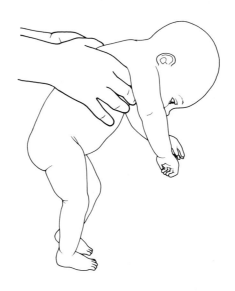

Supported standing (1)

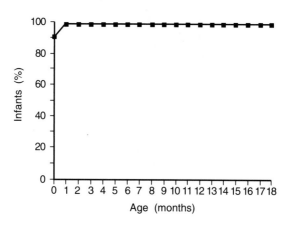

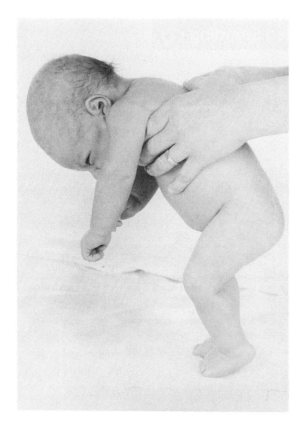

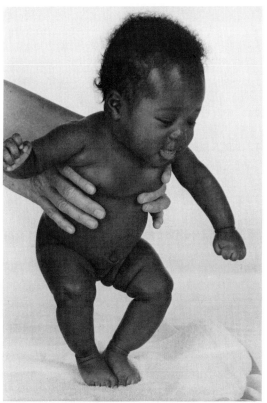

Supported Standing (2)

Weight Bearing	Weight on feet or toes
Posture	Head in line with body Hips behind shoulders Hips flexed and abducted
Antigravity Movement	Variable movement of legs May bend and straighten knees May hyperextend knees May stamp with one foot

The antigravity movements observed in the legs are extremely variable. Some flexion of the legs is observed in the resting posture.

Prompt: The infant is supported by examiner under the axillae.

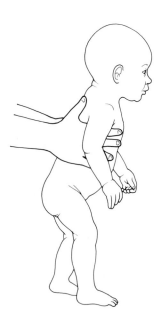

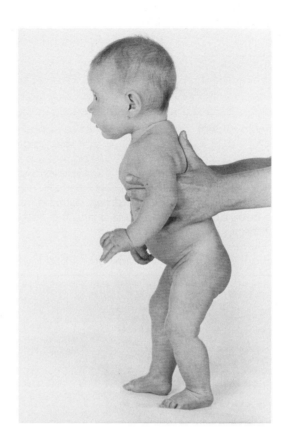

Supported standing (2)

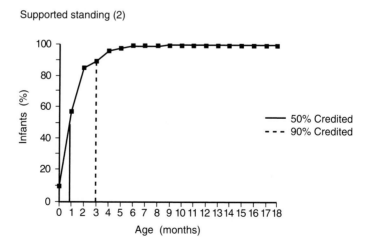

Supported Standing (3)

Weight Bearing	Weight on feet
Posture	Head in midline Hips in line with shoulders Hips abducted and externally rotated
Antigravity Movement	Active control of trunk Variable movements of legs: may bounce up and down, lift one leg, or hyperextend the knees

The antigravity movements are extremely variable. To pass this item, the infant must have the heels down at some point during the observation period and demonstrate spontaneous movement in the legs.

Prompt: Infant is supported by examiner at chest level.

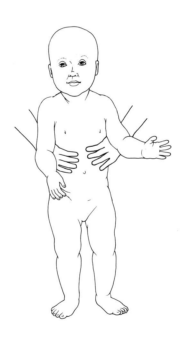

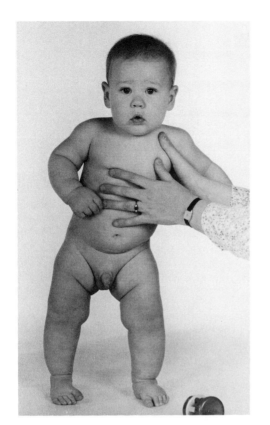 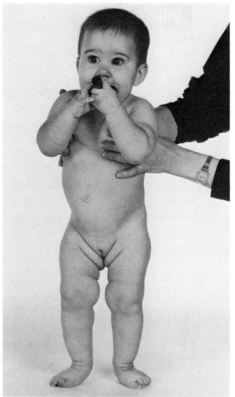

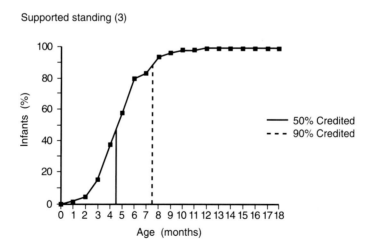

Supported standing (3)

Pulls to Stand with Support

Weight Bearing	Weight on arms and feet
Posture	Arms on support Hips abducted and externally rotated Leans on support Lumbar lordosis
Antigravity Movement	Pushes down with arms and extends knees to achieve standing

The legs do not have to be completely symmetrical during this maneuver, and the infant may push with the legs to assume the position. The posture of the feet is variable; weight bearing may be observed on the toes or medial border of the feet.

Prompt: May use toys to encourage infant to get to standing position. Do not place in standing position.

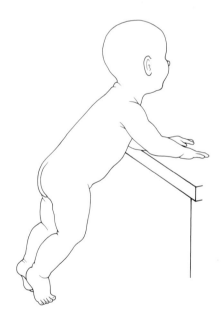

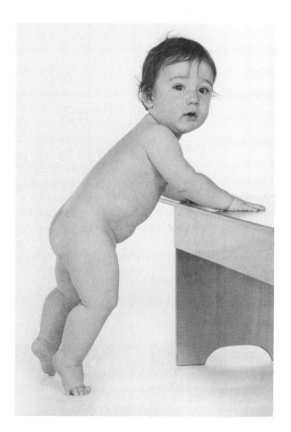

Pulls to stand with support

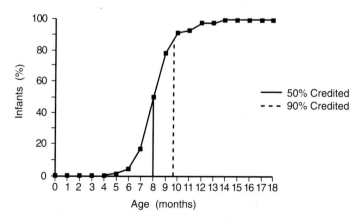

Pulls to Stand/Stands

Weight Bearing	Weight on feet Some arm support
Posture	Hips flexed, abducted, and externally rotated Lumbar lordosis Broad stance
Antigravity Movement	Pulls to stand Shifts weight from side to side May lift one leg off surface No rotation in trunk

The examiner must observe the infant independently assume the standing position. The infant may pull to stand through postures other than half-kneeling.

Prompt: May use toys to encourage infant to stand.

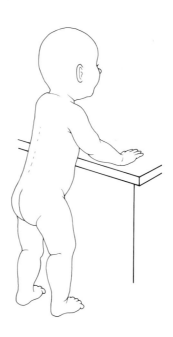

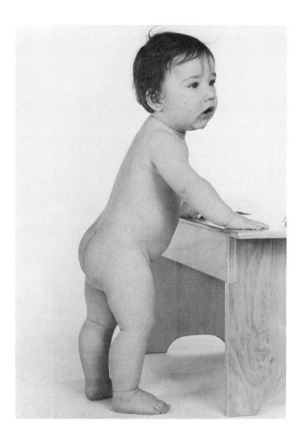

Pulls to stand/stands

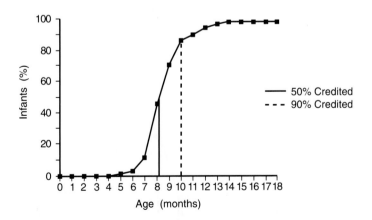

Supported Standing with Rotation

Weight Bearing	Weight on feet One-arm support
Posture	Hips abducted Trunk rotated
Antigravity Movement	Able to release one hand and reach with rotation of trunk and pelvis

If the infant is not observed to pull to stand independently, he or she should not pass this item. The infant's base of support may still be wide.

Prompt: May use toys to elicit trunk rotation.

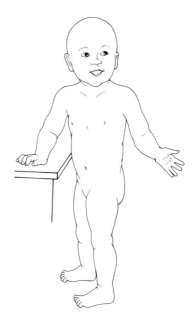

Supported standing with rotation

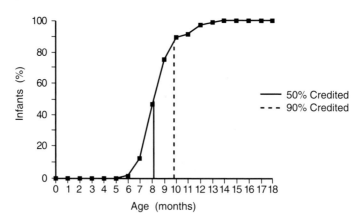

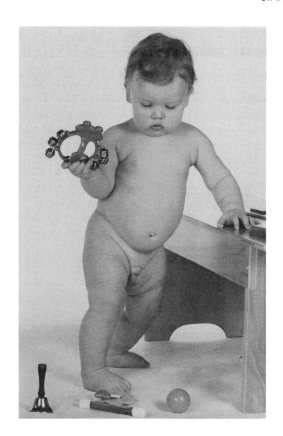

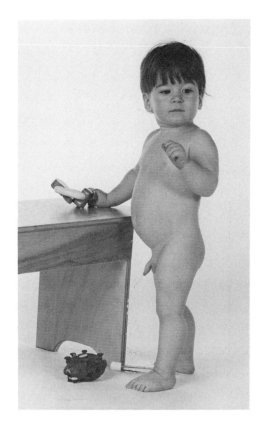

Cruising Without Rotation

Weight Bearing	Weight on feet Some arm support
Posture	Legs abducted and externally rotated Wide base of support
Antigravity Movement	Cruises sideways without rotation

If the infant is not observed to pull to stand independently, he or she should not pass this item. The infant may go up on the toes in standing but should be observed to assume a plantigrade position some of the time.

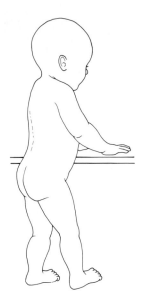

Cruising without rotation

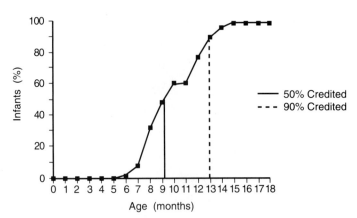

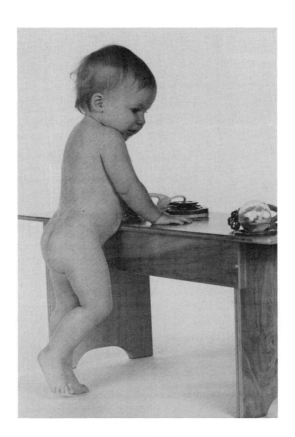

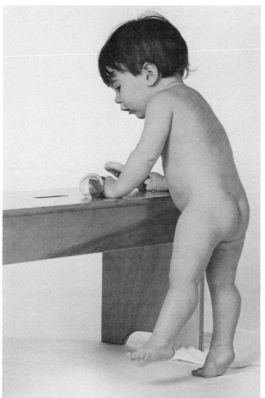

Half-Kneeling

Weight Bearing	Weight on one flexed knee and the opposite foot; arm support
Posture	Half-kneeling posture
Antigravity Movement	May assume standing or play in position

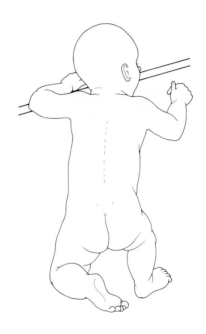

Half-kneeling

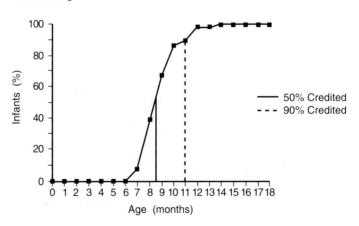

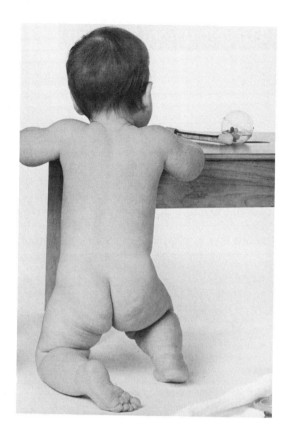

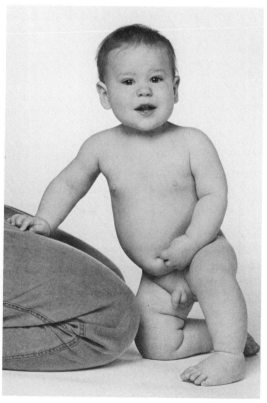

Controlled Lowering from Standing

Weight Bearing	Weight on feet
	One-arm support

Posture	Holds onto support with one hand

Antigravity Movement	Controlled lowering from standing

To pass this item, the infant must assume standing independently. A variety of leg postures may be observed; the legs may move symmetrically or asymmetrically. The movement must be controlled, and the infant must not accidentally fall from the standing position. The infant does not have to return to standing.

Prompt: May use toys to elicit the antigravity movements.

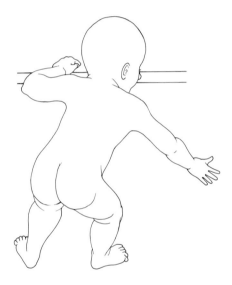

Controlled lowering from standing

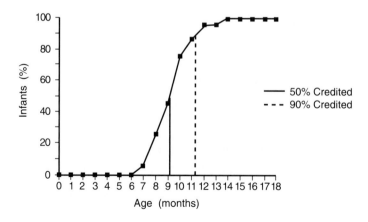

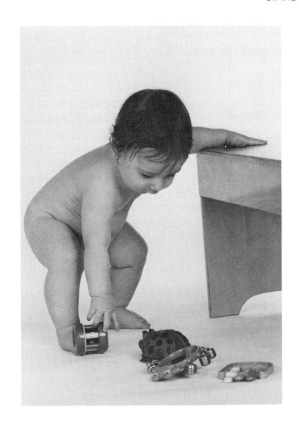

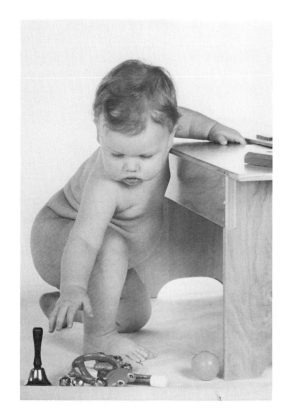

Cruising with Rotation

Weight Bearing	Weight on feet Some arm support
Posture	Semiturned in direction of movement
Antigravity Movement	Cruises with rotation

If the infant is not observed to pull to stand independently, he or she should not pass this item.

Prompt: May use toys to encourage infant to cruise.

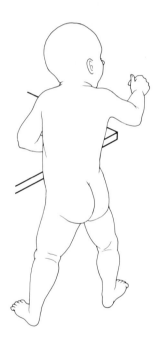

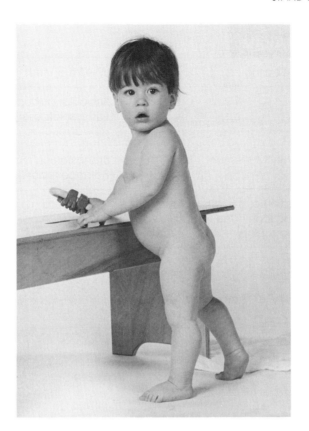

Cruising with rotation

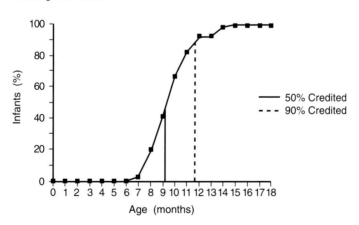

Stands Alone

Weight Bearing	Weight on feet
Posture	Scapular adduction Lumbar lordosis Hips abducted and externally rotated
Antigravity Movement	Stands alone momentarily Balance reactions in feet

The position of the arms may vary from high guard to medium guard position. Balance reactions in the feet can be either dorsiflexion balance reactions or intermittent toe grasping.

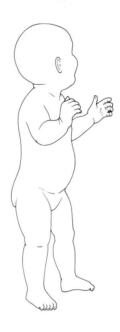

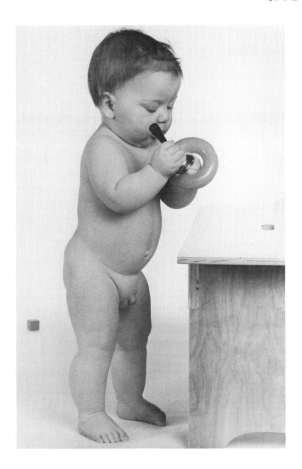

Stands alone

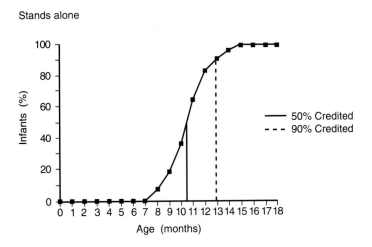

Early Stepping

Weight Bearing	Weight on feet
Posture	Scapular adduction Lumbar lordosis Legs abducted and externally rotated
Antigravity Movement	Walks independently Moves quickly with short steps

The infant must take five independent steps to pass this item. The position of the arms may vary from high guard to medium guard position. This item represents the infant's first attempts to walk independently; he or she may still fall often.

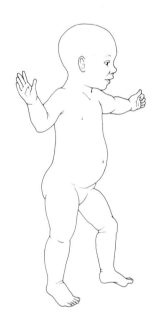

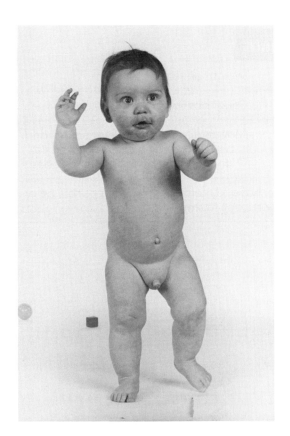
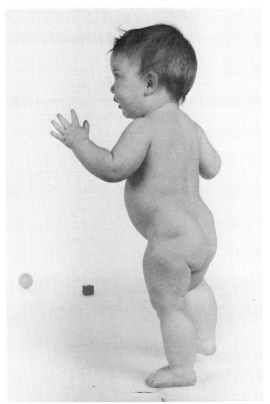

Early stepping

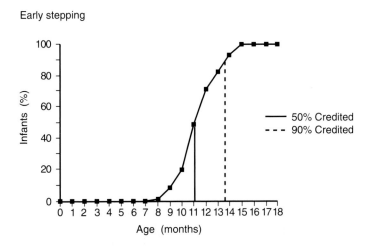

Standing from Modified Squat

Weight Bearing	Weight on feet
Posture	Squat position
Antigravity Movement	Moves from standing to squat and back to standing with controlled flexion and extension of hips and knees

To pass this item, the infant does not have to maintain the squat position; he or she may quickly move from squat position back to standing.

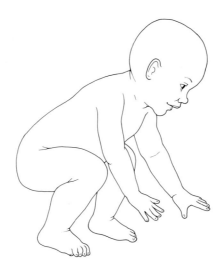

Standing from modified squat

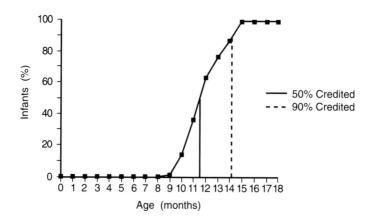

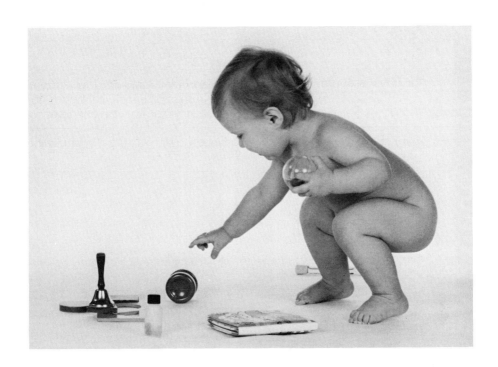

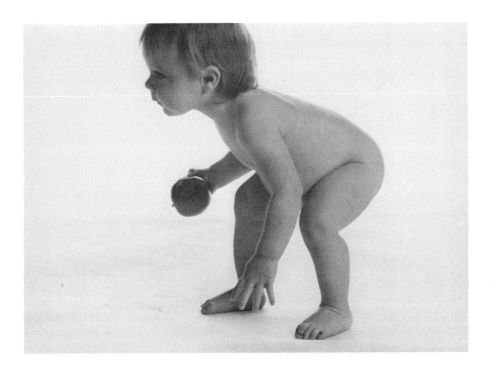

Standing from Quadruped Position

Weight Bearing	Weight on hands and feet
Posture	Hands and feet
Antigravity Movement	Assumes standing independently Pushes quickly with hands to get to standing without using any props

Prompt: To elicit this item, the examiner may position the infant in the supine position and observe the response.

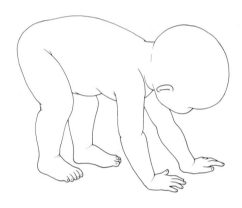

Standing from quadruped position

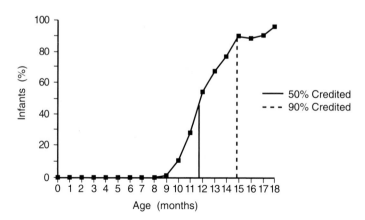

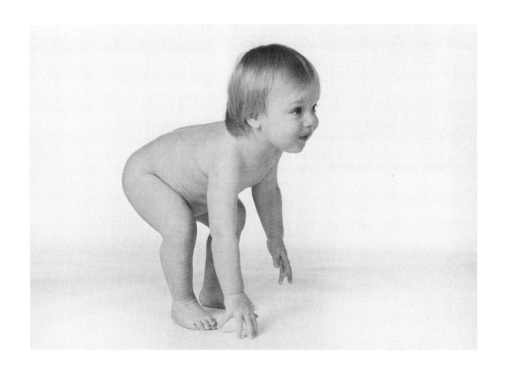

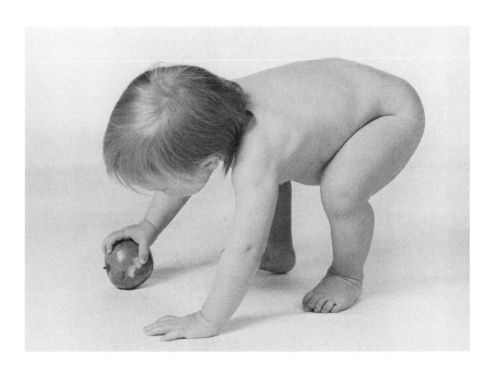

Walks Alone

Weight Bearing	Weight on feet
Posture	Arms may vary from medium guard to low guard to side of body positions Lumbar lordosis Legs neutral or slightly abducted
Antigravity Movement	Walks independently

To pass this item, the infant uses walking as the main method of locomotion. The walking pattern may still be immature.

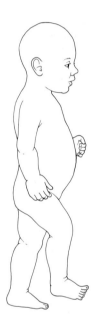

Walks alone

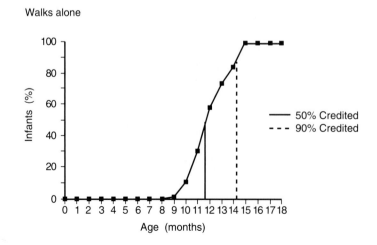

Age (months)

— 50% Credited

--- 90% Credited

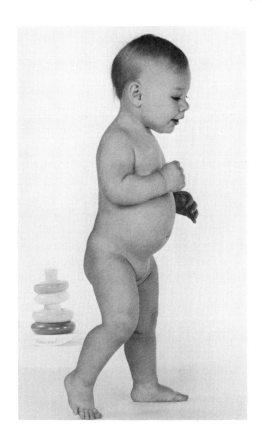

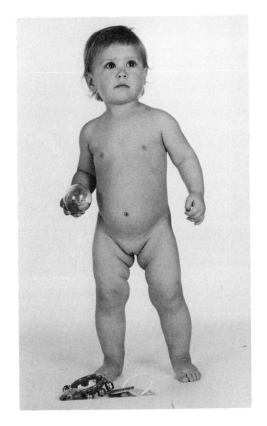

Squat

Weight Bearing	Weight on feet
Posture	Squat posture; trunk forward
Antigravity Movement	Maintains position by balance reactions in feet and position of trunk

The infant is able to play in this position.

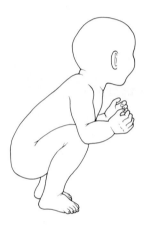

Squat

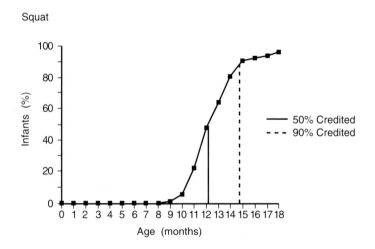

— 50% Credited
- - - 90% Credited

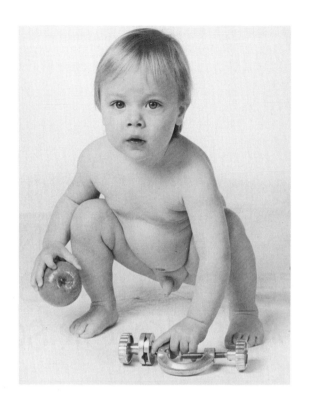

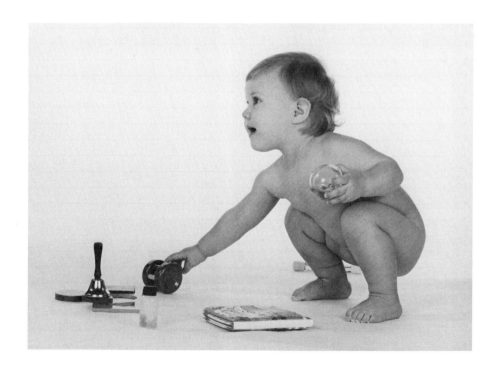

CLINICAL USES OF THE ALBERTA INFANT MOTOR SCALE

Interest in the development of typical and atypical infants has been increasing rapidly over the past decade, thereby resulting in a significant shift in the focus of infant assessments. The expansion of early intervention programs for atypically developing and at-risk infants has shifted the emphasis of infant assessment from long-term prediction to providing information to aid in the planning and execution of intervention activities. Whereas early efforts in infant assessment were aimed at predicting later intellectual or developmental outcomes, infant assessments are now directed at the generation of assessment data to meet the present needs of the infants and their families (Honzik, 1976; McCall, 1979).

This increased attention to the developing infant and infant intervention has led to a rethinking of the specific purposes of infant assessment. Sheehan and Gallagher (1984) suggest that infant assessments now have three essential purposes:

1. These assessments provide a cost-efficient method of reliably *identifying* those infants who are in need of further diagnostic assessment or treatment (Frankenburg, 1975).
2. They provide information for *evaluating* an infant's progress over time, as a result of either maturation or early intervention (Sheehan and Keogh, 1981).
3. Information regarding the infant's strengths and weaknesses is also provided, with the results used as a basis for *planning* intervention strategies (Bricker and Littman, 1982).

The Alberta Infant Motor Scale (AIMS) was constructed to assess the motor development of infants from birth through 18 months of age. Within this context, it was developed to fulfill all of the preceding three purposes: identification, evaluation, and planning.

The AIMS may be used to identify infants who exhibit normal motor development, infants who have normal patterns of movement but demonstrate immature motor skills for their age, and infants who exhibit abnormal patterns of movement suggestive of a specific motor disorder, such as cerebral palsy. The AIMS may also be used to evaluate and monitor changes in the motor development of infants over the first 18 months of life. These changes in motor performance may be the result of maturation or intervention. Because the AIMS is based on normal constructs of movement, its evaluative function should be limited to infants displaying immature motor abilities resulting in motor delay. It is not appropriate to use the AIMS to evaluate the longitudinal changes in motor development of infants exhibiting pathological patterns of movement.

Finally, the AIMS may be used to assist health professionals in planning treatment goals and intervention strategies for at-risk infants or infants with immature motor abilities. Information derived from the AIMS may be used to determine the focus of interventions aimed at facilitating the progression of motor development.

IDENTIFICATION

A discriminative test identifies the *current* performance of individuals on a particular dimension (Kirshner and Guyatt, 1985). Criteria are established defining different levels of performance on the particular domain evaluated. For example, scores on tests of intelligence are used to distinguish different levels of learning abilities; the American Association of Mental Deficiency identifies persons with retardation by using scores on intelligence tests that are approximately 2 SD below the normative sample mean (Anastasi, 1988).

The AIMS evaluates the domain of infant motor development; scores obtained by infants on the AIMS may be used to identify different levels or percentile ranks of motor performance in infants. Through the use of the AIMS, the clinician is appraised of the infant's current motor development status. This appraisal of an infant's motor abilities is accomplished by using the normative data of the AIMS; these data permit the test user to determine the percentile rank of an infant's AIMS score by comparing it with the scores of a sample of age-matched infants. For example, an infant whose score falls below the 5th percentile rank for his or her age group has a score that is lower than 95% of the infants of the same age in the normative sample. This infant's motor abilities are clearly delayed when compared with the majority of infants at a similar age. Within this discriminative role, the AIMS will identify those infants whose motor abilities are immature but exhibit normal patterns of movement, as well as those infants who display abnormal patterns of movement.

Information derived from the AIMS permits the identification of deviations from normal motor development as early as possible in the infant's life. In particular, the AIMS identifies the strengths and weaknesses of the infant's motor performance in regard to motor development norms and expectations. The AIMS, however, is not a diagnostic tool; rather, it must be employed as part of a clinical program in which there is a well-defined plan for using the acquired information. Specifically, when used for the purpose of identification, the AIMS provides the basis for decisions regarding appropriate treatment, ongoing monitoring, or more extensive diagnostic testing.

The results of a discriminative test should not be used to make inferences or predictions about an infant's eventual or long-term motor outcome. The long-term predictive abilities of infant assessment measures have been shown to be at best marginal when used with almost all but the most profoundly involved infants (Sheehan and Gallagher, 1984). In general, infant motor assessments used by physical and occupational therapists to predict later motor outcomes have been disappointing in their ability to classify infants as to their eventual motor outcomes (Deitz et al., 1987; Harris, 1987; Palisano, 1986).

In reviewing the ability of infant assessment tools to reliably predict later developmental status, three conclusions can be made (Sheehan and Gallagher, 1984):

1. The shorter the time between testing periods, the higher the correlations are between the tests.
2. A linear trend is associated with the testing age—that is, the correlation between infant tests and later measures of development increases with increasing infant age at testing (McCall et al., 1977).
3. The predictive capability of infant measures is highly related to the severity index, or stated differently, infant tests are reliable predictors for infants who are functioning at the extreme low end of the developmental continuum (Lewis, 1975; Meier, 1975, 1976). Such low functioning performance in infancy is usually self-evident and does not require formal assessment procedures to be accurately identified (Brooks-Gunn and Lewis, 1981).

For these reasons, the AIMS has a limited role in predicting later motor outcomes when administered either to very young infants or infants who exhibit minor or moderate delays in motor skills. Clearly, as with all infant assessments, the predictive validity of the AIMS should increase with the age of the infant and the severity of the motor delay. The predictive validity of the AIMS when administered to at-risk infants is currently under investigation.

Nevertheless, it is important to understand that an infant who receives a low score on the AIMS will not necessarily remain delayed in subsequent motor development. A single low percentile ranking should not be interpreted in isolation as evidence of future motor delays. Rather the evaluator must use clinical judgment to determine the significance of the current motor delay identified by the infant's AIMS score and decide accordingly on the appropriate clinical action, such as continued follow-up and monitoring, treatment, or more extensive diagnostic testing.

In summary, the AIMS is a useful tool to identify different levels of motor development in infants from birth to 18 months of life. Infants may be assessed in the context of well baby clinics, pediatric office examinations, or neonatal follow-up clinics for infants who are at risk for developmental problems. In each of these settings, the AIMS may assist health care professionals in identifying infants who are currently experiencing difficulty in motor skills in comparison to their age-matched peers. The interpretation of this information will require professional judgment and will be dependent, to some extent, on the age of the infant at the time of the assessment, the severity of the delay, and the patterns of movement exhibited. The clinical actions that might be taken as a result of an identified delay in motor development include ongoing monitoring and follow-up, intervention or treatment aimed at remediating or minimizing the delay, or more extensive diagnostic testing.

EVALUATION

An evaluative index measures changes in an individual's performance over time in a particular ability or skill (Kirshner and Guyatt, 1985). When used to evaluate infant behavior, an evaluative test must be responsive to changes attributable to maturation. Infant growth charts are an example of evaluative indices employed with infants; the charts document the changes in the height and weight of an infant over time. As the infant matures, the height and weight measurements increase and are thus sensitive indicators of the maturational changes of the infant. As such, they serve as a record of the changes occurring in height and weight over time, and any deviances from the expected rates of change can be detected and investigated.

The AIMS may be used to evaluate changes over time in the domain of infant motor development during the first 18 months of life. As an infant ages and matures, new motor skills are mastered, and the AIMS score increases. Thus, the change in an infant's AIMS scores over time may be used as an indicator of the change or maturation of the infant's motor abilities.

Because the AIMS is sensitive to small increments of change over brief periods, it is capable of detecting maturational changes. During the evaluation of the test-retest reliability of the AIMS, changes in scores were obtained over a 1-week period. Two assessments were performed on the same infants within 1 week; analyses of the test scores at the two points in time revealed a difference between the two mean scores, with the second score being consistently higher than the earlier score (see Chapter 10 for more detailed information). Changes in motor abilities over such a brief period can be quite subtle; the fact that the AIMS is able to document these changes suggests that it may be used as a sensitive evaluative index of infant motor development.

This evaluative role may be useful in the surveillance of infant development, a new concept in pediatric care. Pediatricians in both the United States and Britain are advocating surveillance of an infant's development rather than a rigid timetable of assessments and screening (Dworkin, 1989). Dworkin distinguishes surveillance from screening by describing it as a "flexible, continuous process," unlike screening that entails fixed ages for testing (Dworkin, 1989, p 1006). The philosophy of surveillance emphasizes the ongoing observation of an infant's unfolding development by the parent or health professional. Within this model, changes in an infant's score on the AIMS could be used to document an infant's motor development. In addition, both the AIMS score sheet and developmental graph provide an excellent visual history of changes in an infant's motor abilities over time.

As an evaluative index, the AIMS may also be useful to monitor or document changes in infants with immature motor skills who are receiving intervention. Two main goals of therapists treating infants with immature motor skills are to encourage new, age-appropriate motor skills and to foster more mature patterns of movement in the current motor abilities of the infants.

The AIMS is capable of evaluating both of these goals. In addition to outlining the sequence of emergence of new motor skills, the items on the AIMS also chronicle maturational changes that occur within a specific motor skill. For example, in the *prone subscale,* an infant will receive credit if the pattern of reciprocal creeping changes from an immature, wide-based one to a more mature creeping pattern with the hips aligned under the pelvis. It is precisely these qualitative, maturational changes in motor skills that physical and occupational therapists strive to affect with treatment. Current infant motor tests have proved unsatisfactory in detecting these changes in motor skills (Campbell, 1991).

Motor tests such as the Peabody Gross and Fine Motor Scales (Folio and Fewell, 1983) attempt to capture maturational changes within a specific skill by using time and distance as indicators of improvement. Conversely, the AIMS describes the changes occurring in the components of the movement. Because the AIMS captures both the changes across motor skills and the changes within a motor skill due to maturation, it may be a valuable tool for assessing the changes that occur as a result of intervention. Further research is required to substantiate this claim. In addition, the methodological dilemma of isolating the changes resulting from intervention from the changes associated with maturation remains.

PLANNING

Most of the current interest in infant assessment is directed toward the purpose of planning intervention strategies for delayed or at-risk infants (Kaiser and Hayden, 1977). Stowers and Huber (1987) suggest that the results obtained from infant assessments are useful for designing intervention programs. Much of the teaching that goes on with infants having delayed motor skills is drawn directly from developmental measures. As Kaiser and Hayden note, "Special educators try to facilitate the progression of infants with developmental delays through normal learning sequences that most babies go through naturally" (Kaiser and Hayden, 1977, p 9).

Because the focus of the AIMS is on the sequential development of motor skills coupled with the emphasis on the components of movement, the AIMS is ideally suited to assist therapists in identifying a framework for their intervention strategies. Each AIMS item is described according to three components: (1) the part of the body that bears weight, (2) the posture of the infant, and (3) the antigravity movements an infant must demonstrate in order to receive credit for the item. Thus, each item provides an analysis of the essential components of the motor skill necessary for an infant to successfully accomplish the item. In addition, the AIMS assessment cues the therapist as to which motor skills the infant has already achieved and the next skills in the anticipated motor sequence.

When an infant is identified as being delayed in motor abilities and is referred for treatment, the therapist can examine the infant's performance on the AIMS as recorded on the score sheet and readily identify the "not observed" items in the infant's current motor "window." By reviewing the written descriptions of the criteria necessary to pass these items, the therapist is provided with a framework to examine the components of the skill that the infant is currently unable to accomplish. Knowledge of these missing components enables the therapist to design a treatment program that will introduce the missing components into the infant's motor repertoire. For example, if an infant is unable to maintain the head above 45° when in the prone position, the therapist can determine from the description of this item that to success-

TABLE 9–1
Clinical Uses of the AIMS

Purpose of the Assessment	Characteristics of Infants to Be Assessed		
	Normal	Immature Motor Skills	Abnormal Patterns of Movement
Identification of motor delays	+	+	+
Evaluation of change over time	+	+	−
Treatment planning	NA	+	+

fully accomplish this skill, the infant must bear weight on the upper chest, and the elbows must be at least in line with the shoulders. This information provides a focus for the treatment planned by the therapist. This feature of the AIMS may be especially valuable to therapists who are less experienced and who have not had the opportunity to observe normally developing infants. Although the AIMS is not intended to provide "cookbook" solutions for the treatment of infants with motor delays, it may assist therapists in identifying the missing components of a motor skill and act as a reference point for the formulation of intervention strategies.

CONCLUSIONS

The AIMS has been constructed to fulfill three clinical purposes of infant motor assessment: the identification of different levels of motor performance, the evaluation of change in motor performance over time resulting from maturation or intervention, and the provision of useful information for the planning of motor intervention strategies. Because the long-term predictive accuracy of the AIMS has yet to be determined, it is inappropriate at this time to employ the AIMS as a predictive index.

The applicability of the AIMS to different groups of infants is largely determined by the purpose of the assessment. For example, the AIMS should not be used to evaluate changes in motor development over time with infants having abnormal patterns of movement. Table 9–1 summarizes the clinical uses of the AIMS in terms of the groups of infants who may be appropriately assessed given the specific focus of the assessment.

In conclusion, the purpose of the assessment and the characteristics of the infants being assessed will determine the clinical applicability and interpretation of the scores derived from the AIMS. Although the AIMS has been developed to fulfill several clinical functions, it needs to be applied differentially according to the objectives of the assessment and the infant's patterns of movement.

References

Anastasi A: *Psychological Testing,* 6th ed. New York, Macmillan, 1988.

Bricker D, Littman D: Intervention and evaluation: the inseparable mix. Top Early Child Spec Educ 1982;2(4):23–34.

Brooks-Gunn J, Lewis M: Assessing young handicapped children: issues and solutions. J Div Early Child 1981;2:84–95.

Campbell SK: Framework for the measurement of neurologic impairment and disability. In: *Contemporary Management of Motor Control Problems.* Proceedings of the II STEP Conference. Alexandria VA, Foundation for Physical Therapy, 1991, pp 143–154.

Deitz JC, Crowe TK, Harris SR: Relationship

between infant neuromotor assessment and preschool motor measures. Phys Ther 1987;67(1):14–17.

Dworkin PH: British and American recommendations for developmental monitoring: the role of surveillance. Pediatrics 1989; 84(6):1000–1010.

Folio MR, Fewell RR: *Peabody Developmental Motor Scales and Activity Cards: A Manual.* Allen TX, DLM Teaching Resources, 1983.

Frankenburg WK: Criteria in screening test selection. In: Frankenburg WK, Camp BW (eds): *Pediatric Screening Tests.* Springfield, IL, Charles C Thomas, 1975, pp 23–37.

Harris SR: Early detection of cerebral palsy: sensitivity and specificity of two motor assessment tools. J Perinatol 1987;7(1):11–15.

Honzik MP: Value and limitations of infant tests: an overview. In: Lewis M (ed): *Origins of Intelligence.* New York, Plenum Press, 1976, pp 59–95.

Kaiser C, Hayden A: The education of the very, very young or but what can you teach an infant? Educ Horiz 1977;56(1):4–15.

Kirshner B, Guyatt G: A methodological framework for assessing health and disease. J Chron Dis 1985;38:27–36.

Lewis M: The development of attention and perception in the infant and young child. In: Cruickshank WM, Hallahan DP (eds): *Perceptual and Learning Disabilities in Children,* vol 2. Syracuse NY, Syracuse University Press, 1975, pp 137–162.

McCall RB: The development of intellectual functioning in infancy and the prediction of later I.Q. In: Osofsky JD (ed): *Handbook of Infant Development.* New York, Wiley, 1979, pp 707–741.

McCall RB, Eichorn DH, Hogarty PS: Transitions in early mental development. Monogr Soc Res Child Dev 1977;42(3):1–13.

Meier JH: Screening, assessment and intervention for young children at developmental risk. In: Hobbs N (ed): *Issues in the Classification of Children,* vol 2. San Francisco, Jossey-Bass, 1975, pp 497–543.

Meier JH: Screening, assessment and intervention for young children at developmental risk. In: Tjossem TD (ed): *Intervention Strategies for High-Risk Infants and Young Children.* Baltimore, University Park Press, 1976, pp 251–287.

Palisano RJ: Concurrent and predictive validities of the Bayley motor scale and the Peabody developmental motor scales. Phys Ther 1986;66(11):1714–1719.

Sheehan R, Gallagher RJ: Assessment of infants. In: Hanson M (ed): *Atypical Infant Development.* Baltimore, University Park Press, 1984, pp 81–106.

Sheehan R, Keogh B: Design and analysis in the evaluation of early childhood special education programs. Top Early Child Spec Educ 1981;1(4):81–88.

Stowers S, Huber CJ: Developmental and screening tests. In: King-Thomas L, Hacker BJ (eds): *A Therapist's Guide to Pediatric Assessment.* Boston, Little, Brown, 1987, pp 43–142.

ten

PSYCHOMETRIC PROPERTIES OF THE AIMS

Lynn Redfern, Ph.D., and Thomas O. Maguire, Ph.D.

An important component of the development of any new instrument is the examination of its reliability and validity. Reliability can be defined as the consistency or reproducibility of scores obtained when the same group of individuals is assessed more than once with the same instrument. In the case of the Alberta Infant Motor Scale (AIMS), it was particularly important to document the reliability among different therapists when assessing the same infant and the reliability of scores obtained at two different points in time.

The validity of an instrument is the adequacy with which it measures the construct of interest. Although reliability is an essential aspect of validity, its presence is not sufficient evidence that the instrument covers the construct of interest—in this case, gross motor maturity. Assessment of validity should be thought of as a process whereby the instrument is subjected to investigations of its concurrent, structural, and discriminant characteristics. The concurrent validity of the AIMS was examined by comparing it to two widely used infant motor scales: the *motor scale* of the Bayley Scales of Infant Development (Bayley, 1969) and the *gross motor scale* of the Peabody Developmental Motor Scales (Folio and Fewell, 1983). Structural validity was examined through an analysis of the dimensionality and other scale properties of the AIMS and by documenting the ability of the instrument to discriminate between normal and abnormal development (the discriminant validity results are reported in Chapter 11).

SAMPLE AND DESIGN

The reliability and validity assessments were performed using data from 506 normal infants recruited through the Edmonton Board of Health well baby clinics and meeting the following inclusion criteria:

Gestational age of 38 to 42 weeks at the time of birth
Birth weight of greater than 2500 g

Uncomplicated delivery
Deemed normal upon discharge from hospital
No obvious abnormality at the time of assessment

The sample size was largely determined by the total number of items in the instrument, which is 58. A sample of approximately 500 infants was believed to be a reasonable compromise between a sufficient number of subjects to conduct a factor analysis and the costs of testing each infant.

The sample was age-stratified, by month, through the first 18 months of life. The upper age limit of 18 months was chosen to be reasonably certain of capturing the age of independent walking in all normal infants. The instrument was constructed with the intent that it would be most sensitive around the middle of the first year of life, since that is generally considered to be the optimal time to identify infants who have a motor delay and to commence treatment programs for them. For this reason, slightly larger numbers of children were sampled in the age categories between 3 and 12 months than in the very young or older age categories.

Data were collected over a period of 15 months, beginning in December 1989 and ending in March 1991. Infants were assessed by one of six pediatric physical therapists who were experienced in infant motor assessment and trained in the administration of the AIMS.

The types of reliability and validity examined included interrater and test-retest reliability, concurrent validity with the Peabody and Bayley motor scales, and an extensive analysis of the scale properties of the new instrument. Thus the design required that some infants be tested by more than one rater and also tested on a second occasion. In addition, certain infants were simultaneously tested on the AIMS, the Peabody *motor scale,* and the Bayley *motor scale.* For the analysis of the instrument's scale properties, only one of these assessments was used, and in each case it was the initial AIMS assessment by the primary rater.

SCALE PROPERTIES OF THE AIMS

The scaling methods, which included tests of dimensionality and procedures for positioning items on the developmental continuum, were carried out with data from 479 infants who ranged in age from 0 to 15 months. Although the sample consisted of infants up to 18 months of age (n = 506), essentially all of the older infants had passed every item. As Wohlwill (1973) points out, "The scalability of any response matrix can be arbitrarily enhanced by ensuring a sufficiently large number of cases of subjects responding to or passing either all or none of the items, which necessarily constitute perfect scale patterns." He further indicates that this problem is most severe in the study of developmental sequences that concern only a limited portion of an age continuum. It was hoped that restricting the sample to only those infants expected to have some mixture of pass-fail scores would minimize this problem.

Tests of Dimensionality

Multidimensional scaling was the primary method for assessing the dimensionality of the data set. This was performed using a nonmetric procedure with ALSCAL (Young et al., 1978). The distance measure selected in the creation of the dissimilarities matrix for input into ALSCAL was the Euclidean distance for binary items. Goodness of fit indices were Kruskal's stress value and the squared correlation between distances and dissimilarities. In accordance with Wohlwill's (1973) recommendation that dimensionality be tested both across and within age levels, multidimensional scaling was applied first to all data from infants 0 to 15 months of age and then to data from several individual age groups.

The multidimensional scaling results, using data from all 479 infants, indicated that a single dimension provides an excellent fit to these data, as evidenced by a stress value of .04 and RSQ of .995. In order to determine the nature of this dimension, the item scale values for the one-dimensional solution were examined in relation to the item order that was expected as a result of the content validation work and the feasibility study. With a few minor exceptions, the scale values for the one-dimensional solution were ordered in the manner expected. This suggests that the dimension is a developmental sequencing one and that the single construct underlying these data is gross motor maturity.

There was some concern that the one-dimensional model may have fit as well as it did because of the large variation in motor ability across the sample strata and the concomitant large variability across the item set in terms of the level of maturity required to perform the behaviors. Nunnally (1978) cautions that it is easy to fool oneself into believing that a unidimensional scale is present when one takes a set of items widely dispersed in difficulty and administers them to a very diverse population. Also, Wohlwill (1973) emphasizes the importance of testing dimensionality both within and across age levels. For these reasons, the analyses were repeated using data within 3-month age groupings of infants.

The stress values for the one-dimensional solution ranged from .054 to .178, slightly higher than that obtained using all 479 infants. This finding probably reflects the fact that age (i.e., maturity) was the largest contributor to the variation among item scores. Grouping the data by age category removed much of the influence of age, with the result that the variance among items within age groups appears somewhat less systematic.

Still, for the majority of age groups, the stress values for the one-dimensional solution were very close to the two-dimensional stress values, which ranged from .003 to .106. Thus the conclusion that the scale is unidimensional was still deemed reasonable.

Dimensionality was also examined through nonlinear factor analysis, using the program NOHARM (Fraser and McDonald, 1988). The fit of a one-factor model was excellent, as determined by item loadings of 1 or near 1 on the single factor, very small unique variances, and a root mean square of residuals of .0174. Comparison with a two-factor nonlinear model was carried out by applying the Incremental Fit Index (De Champlain and Gessaroli, 1991). This involves comparing the residuals from the one-factor solution to the residuals from the two-factor solution. In this case, the fit index was zero, providing further strong evidence of unidimensionality.

Methods for Positioning Items

Nonmetric multidimensional scaling was the first model applied for the purposes of scaling the items, since it allowed the option of scaling on as many dimensions as were found to be necessary to adequately fit the data. The nonmetric approach had the advantage of producing scale values with interval level properties, while requiring only ordinal level assumptions about the relationships in the original data.

A second approach to item scaling was to examine item difficulty estimates derived according to various models. The method used first was a simple calculation of the proportion of infants passing each item, and this was obtained using the program LERTAP (Nelson, 1974). Next, a two-parameter item response model was applied to the data using the program LOGIST (Wingersky et al., 1982), and the item difficulty estimates were obtained.

Item difficulty estimates were then obtained from the NOHARM nonlinear factor analysis results. Further evidence as to the sequencing of items, as well as the actual distance between items on the age continuum, was gathered by examining the age at which 50% of infants passed each particular item. It was clear that the positioning of items was very similar, regardless of the scaling method used, and this provided convincing evidence of the validity of the item sequence.

Because the various models tested suggested almost identical item sequences, practical considerations such as ease of application and interpretability became the criteria for selecting a scaling model. By these criteria, multidimensional scaling seemed the most useful and so was used to position the items on the final version of the AIMS.

SCORING SYSTEM

Following the determination of item sequence, the infants' test scores were derived according to two different scoring systems:

1. "Pass" scores were summed for each infant, giving a total number of items passed (range of 1 to 58).
2. Items were reordered, based on their multidimensional scale values, and a score was given to each infant corresponding to the position (1 to 58) of the highest item passed.

Each of these scoring systems had a certain appeal to the members of the research team. The "number of items passed" is the system used with most well-known motor scales and is very straightforward in its calculation. It also lends itself quite easily to the construction of norms tables, since typical total scores and ranges (or percentiles) can be reported for various age groups of infants. A total score or percentile rank is generally considered to be less problematic than certain other types of scores such as age equivalents, particularly when reporting an infant's performance to the parents.

The "highest item passed" system possesses the same advantages with regard to calculation, norming, and reporting. However, it has the added appeal of being a compensatory model for scoring, since it gives an infant credit for the level at which he or she is currently capable of performing, regardless of which behaviors were or were not performed previously. Thus the use of this system would avoid the situation of awarding "pass" scores for behaviors not actually observed but assumed to have been performed at an earlier time. It is also consistent with the opinion of many experts in infant motor assessment that it is the endpoint that is important in determining an infant's motor ability, rather than the means by which the infant arrived at that endpoint.

In order to evaluate the two scoring systems quantitatively, both types of scores were computed for all 506 infants. The correlation between the two scores was found to be .99, indicating a high degree of consistency across these two systems, when applied to data from normal infants. In addition, the infant's age had a strong relationship both with "number of items passed" (r = .95) and "highest item passed" (r = .94). These findings provided no real basis for choosing one scoring method over the other.

Through discussions within the research team, it was recognized that the consistency observed between the scoring methods might not hold when the instrument was applied to high-risk or abnormal infants. Specifically, it was felt that abnormal infants might pass certain items but be incapable of performing some earlier behaviors, particularly in a different postural position. This could give such an infant a higher score than was appropriate if scoring was based upon the highest item passed. For this reason, it was decided that the total number of items passed was a more reasonable scoring system to retain.

RELIABILITY

Overview

The reliability of the AIMS was examined in two ways. Two hundred and fifty-three infants were examined by two trained therapist assessors simultaneously. One of the assessors was designated as the "primary" assessor and was responsible for carrying out the actual assessment. The other assessor, the "observer" assessor, took a more passive role and observed the assessment as it proceeded, scoring the result independently of the first therapist. Comparison of the scores gives an indication of interassessor stability at one time.

From 3 to 7 days later, a second assessment was scheduled for each infant. In about one third of the cases, this second assessment was done by a therapist who had not been involved either as primary assessor or observer with that infant. In about one third of the cases, the primary assessor made the reassessment, and in the final third of the cases, the observer assessor was used. Comparisons of the scores for the first analysis provide evidence about the joint effects of time and rater differences on the stability of ratings. The other two data sets give an indication of the effects of time on the stability of ratings. Because the infants' abilities change fairly rapidly, the influences of time are confounded with true growth or development. The time interval chosen was a compromise between making the time long enough so that the results of the first assessment would not influence the second to a great extent and the need to keep the interval short enough so that the infants' motor development had not changed substantially. In all, six assessors participated in the reliability study. Their involvement as primary, observer, and follow-up assessors was counterbalanced. However, to keep scheduling manageable, they were divided into two teams of three individuals. The assessment plan is shown in Table 10–1 for one of the teams. Approximately 40 infants did not return for the follow-up assessment.

The results were examined in several ways. Since the total score on the AIMS is used to estimate infant motor development, the main focus of the analyses was to provide estimates of reliability for total scores, both across and within age levels. Infants were selected for the reliability study to provide

TABLE 10–1
Reliability Plan

	Time 1	Time 2	Type
	Ab	C	3
	Ab	A	1
	Ac	B	3
	Ac	C	2
	Ba	C	3
	Ba	A	2
	Bc	A	3
	Bc	B	1
	Ca	B	3
	Ca	C	1
	Cb	A	3
	Cb	B	2

A, B, C = primary assessor; a, b, c = observer assessor; type 1 = primary rater over time; type 2 = observer rater over time; type 3 = different rater—different time.

representation from birth to 17 months. For the purposes of these analyses, the age groups were clustered into four levels: birth through 3 months, 4 through 7 months, 8 through 11 months, and 12 months or older. There are two aspects to reliability that are important in the present context. First, the correlation between assessments should be high, and second, the difference between the means of the two sets of observations should be very small.

Interrater Reliabilities on One Occasion

The sample sizes, means, standard deviations, and correlations for total AIMS scores are shown in Table 10–2 for the total group and for each of the four age groups.

For the total score, the correlations between observers on a single occasion are very high, and the difference between the means of primary and observing assessors is very small. The standard error of measurement is about one item. In short, the instrument is very stable over raters at one time. Of course, the correlation for total scores is aided by the developmental trend that runs through the scale as shown in the various dimensional analyses. To see how stable the instrument is at various age levels, reliabilities and standard errors were calculated at each of the four levels. The lowest correlations occurred for the youngest and oldest children who are actually observed doing the fewest number of items. However, even here the reliabilities exceed .95. The reliabilities translate into standard errors of about 1 point for the youngest age group and for the infants in the 8- to 11-month-old group. The 4- to 7-month-old

TABLE 10–2
Interrater Reliability Data for a Single Occasion

Sample	Primary Mean	Observer Mean	Primary SD	Observer SD	SE	Reliability	Sample Size
Total	34.73	34.66	18.65	18.63	1.01	.9967	253
0–3 mo	10.12	9.93	4.26	4.07	0.86	.9556	56
4–7 mo	26.57	26.65	8.05	8.00	1.38	.9699	81
8–11 mo	48.56	48.37	8.26	8.32	1.11	.9822	62
12 mo +	56.61	56.57	2.30	2.05	0.41	.9588	54

TABLE 10–3
Interrater Reliability Data Across Occasions

Sample	First Mean	Second Mean	First SD	Second SD	SE	Reliability	Sample Size
One occasion	34.73	34.66	18.65	18.63	1.01	.9967	253
Type 1	34.95	35.93	19.81	19.81	1.32	.9556	56
Type 2	33.21	33.98	18.04	18.04	1.57	.9925	56
Type 3	33.78	35.31	18.67	18.26	1.92	.9891	98

group has a standard error of about 1.4 items, and the oldest group has a standard error of 0.45. What all of this means in practical terms is that trained assessors can be used interchangeably to assess infants without increasing the error of measurement to an important extent.

Interrater Reliabilities over Time

In Table 10–3, the reliabilities are shown for raters over time. For comparison purposes, the interassessor values for the total group are reproduced from Table 10–2. Type 1 reliabilities are based on the *primary* assessor being used on both occasions, type 2 reliabilities involve the *observing* assessor being used on both occasions, and type 3 reliabilities involve an assessor who had not previously seen the infant being used on the second occasion.

For the three types of reliabilities calculated over time, the mean for the second occasion is about one item higher than the mean for the first occasion. Since the correlations are very high, it seems likely that the difference in means is largely due to real changes in infant performance. The differences between type 1 and type 2 reliability information is so small that for subsequent analyses no distinction was made between whether the rater at the first assessment was a primary or secondary assessor. The standard error of measurement that includes both occasion variation and between-rater variation is equivalent to about two items. Because it is larger than the values for types 1 and 2, it was decided to examine the effects of different raters over time for each of the age levels.

No distinction is made between primary and observer raters in Table 10–4, in which the results of the reliability analysis are presented for the effect of one rater on two occasions separated by up to 1 week. The results of the total sample are repeated to make comparisons easier.

The trend found in the total sample in which the second mean is about one item higher than the first mean continues with some variation at all age levels. This could be true growth coupled with the effect of the infant becoming

TABLE 10–4
Interrater Reliability Data Over Time (Same Assessor at Both Times)

Sample	First Mean	Second Mean	First SD	Second SD	SE	Reliability	Sample Size
Total	34.08	34.95	12.89	12.87	1.12	.9925	112
0–3 mo	10.11	10.92	3.81	3.60	0.84	.9485	26
4–7 mo	24.95	26.31	5.54	5.64	1.55	.9230	36
8–11 mo	49.87	50.51	7.68	7.19	1.11	.9775	25
12 mo +	56.36	56.84	1.43	1.36	0.53	.8585	25

TABLE 10–5
Interrater Reliability Data Over Time (Different Assessor at Both Times)

Sample	First Mean	Second Mean	First SD	Second SD	SE	Reliability	Sample Size
Total	33.78	35.31	18.67	18.26	1.92	.9891	98
0–3 mo	9.12	10.08	3.43	3.48	1.42	.8245	24
4–7 mo	28	30.70	7.58	7.99	1.95	.9267	30
8–11 mo	46.80	47.64	8.79	8.88	2.24	.9352	25
12 mo +	56.36	56.89	1.79	2.18	0.74	.8634	19

more accustomed to the test setting on the second occasion. The reliabilities are all high except for the 25 infants in the oldest age group. Here, the infants are actually responding to relatively few items. For example, in the oldest age group the test is, in effect, a test of the standing items. Consequently, the shortness of the instrument for the oldest group accounts for part of the relatively low reliability. The high means for the oldest infants arise from the scoring that assumes that the infant can perform (or could have performed) skills in the prone, supine, and sitting positions.

The results of the reliability study that confounds time with different assessors is shown in Table 10–5. Here the raters on each occasion are seeing the child for the first time.

Once again, the second observation results are generally higher than the first. The differences are slightly larger than those observed when the same rater was used over two times. At all ages, except the odd result at 4 to 7 months, the differences between raters over time were less than one item. The 2.7-item difference at 4 to 7 months does not yield to any simple explanation. The standard errors calculated in Table 10–5 are larger than those found in Table 10–4. These differences should be treated cautiously given the small sample sizes.

In interpreting scores at different age levels for a single administration of the AIMS, it might be useful to take the infant's observed score and add and subtract 1 standard error from it. This will produce an approximate 67% confidence band on the raw scores. Looking up the two ends of the confidence band on the table of percentiles provides an indication of how much the infant's score (expressed in percentile units) might be expected to vary from rater to rater. The results of using a confidence band may inject a healthy note of caution in the interpretation.

CONCURRENT VALIDITY

For the concurrent validity component, infants' total scores on the AIMS were correlated with the Peabody Developmental Motor Scales' *gross motor* raw scores and with the *motor scale* of the Bayley Scales of Infant Development raw scores. These two scales were selected because they are the most widely used standardized infant motor scales. Although the limitations of these tools are widely recognized, it was seen as important to report how the new instrument compares with these established scales. Initially, it was anticipated that there would be a midrange correlation between the AIMS and each of these other scales. Very low correlations would be questionable because all three instruments are directed toward the general construct of emerging motor development. Similarly, very high correlations were not antic-

TABLE 10–6
Concurrent Validity (Normal Infants)—Correlation Coefficients

0 to <13 months (n = 103):	
AIMS with Peabody	.99
AIMS with Bayley	.97
Peabody with Bayley	.98
0 to <4 months (n = 23):	
AIMS with Peabody	.90
AIMS with Bayley	.84
Peabody with Bayley	.93
4 to <8 months (n = 37):	
AIMS with Peabody	.98
AIMS with Bayley	.93
Peabody with Bayley	.91
8 to <13 months (n = 43):	
AIMS with Peabody	.94
AIMS with Bayley	.85
Peabody with Bayley	.92

ipated because the new instrument should provide more detailed information than either of the other two assessment scales.

One hundred and twenty infants were assessed by the same therapist on each of the three instruments. Only the 103 infants who were less than 13 months of age were included in the final analysis, since that is the typical age of independent walking, which represents the endpoint of the AIMS. Also, items beyond 13 months on the other two instruments capture behaviors not included within the AIMS, so validation against these more mature items was inappropriate.

Concurrent validity with the two established instruments was estimated with Pearson product-moment correlations, calculated first on all infants less than 13 months of age and then for three individual age groups. The correlations were as shown in Table 10–6.

Concurrent validity with both the *motor scale* of the Bayley Scales of Infant Development and the *gross motor scale* of the Peabody Developmental Motor Scales was also evaluated using 68 abnormal and at-risk infants. The sampling for this analysis is described in Chapter 11. The respective correlation coefficients are listed in Table 10–7.

The magnitude of these correlations, both for the total group and within each age group, and for the normal and abnormal infants, suggests very strong concurrent validity with the other two instruments. Given the evidence that all three instruments measure the same construct, one might question the need for a new instrument for assessing infant motor development. However, the ease of administration of the AIMS, along with the benefits of having a strictly observational assessment method, indicate that this instrument will meet a need not currently being met by existing instruments.

TABLE 10–7
Concurrent Validity (Abnormal and At-risk Infants)—Correlation Coefficients

	Abnormal and At-risk (n = 68)	Abnormal (n = 20)	At-risk (n = 48)
Bayley	.93	.84	.98
Peabody	.95	.87	.98

CONCLUSIONS

The reliability and validity of the AIMS were examined following a thorough analysis of data collected on 506 Edmonton infants. It was concluded that the AIMS is a highly reliable instrument when used by different trained therapists and when applied to the same infants on two different occasions. In addition, there was compelling evidence that the instrument measures a single construct, gross motor maturity, and that its 58 items are appropriately sequenced along the developmental continuum. The high degree of congruence between AIMS scores and the Peabody and Bayley Infant Motor scores provided further evidence that the AIMS is a reliable and valid instrument for the measurement of infant motor development.

References

Bayley N: *Bayley Scales of Infant Development*. Berkeley, Institute of Human Development, University of California, 1969.

De Champlain AD, Gessaroli ME: Assessing Test Dimensionality Using an Index Based on Nonlinear Factor Analysis. Paper presented at the American Educational Research Association Meeting, Chicago, IL, 1991.

Folio MR, Fewell RR: *Peabody Developmental Motor Scales and Activity Cards: A Manual*. Allen TX, DLM Teaching Resources, 1983.

Fraser C, McDonald RP: NOHARM: Least squares item factor analysis. Multivariate Behav Res 1988; 23:267–269.

Nelson LR: *Guide to LERTAP Use and Design* computer program manual. Dunedin, New Zealand, University of Otago, Education Department, 1974.

Nunnally JC: *Psychometric Theory*. New York, McGraw-Hill, 1978.

Wingersky MS, Barton MA, Ford FM: *Logist User's Guide*. Princeton, Educational Testing Service, 1982.

Wohlwill JF: *The Study of Behavioral Development*. New York, Academic Press, 1973.

Young FW, Takane Y, Lewyckyj Y: ALSCAL: a nonmetric multidimensional scaling program with several differences options. Behav Res Methods Instrumentation 1978; 10:451–453.

eleven

NORM-REFERENCING OF THE ALBERTA INFANT MOTOR SCALE

Normative data provide details of the performance of the general population or specific populations so that an individual's performance may be compared with these norms (American Psychological Association, 1983). Because the AIMS was developed to identify those infants who exhibit delayed motor development, normative data are required to determine the individual infant's position with reference to a representative group of infants.

As a result of the provision of norms to aid in the interpretation of individual scores, the AIMS is a norm-referenced test. When additional interpretive data are lacking, a raw score on any test is meaningless. Norm-referenced test interpretation involves some method of examining how an individual's raw test score compares with the scores of others in some similar group.

In the case of the AIMS, the individual infant's test performance is interpreted by comparing it with the performance of a known group of age-matched Albertan infants. This known group is called the *normative sample*. The norms for the AIMS are recorded in a form of a table of equivalents between the *raw scores* (total AIMS score) and the *derived score* (percentile rank). The norms have been empirically established by determining how the infants in the normative sample scored on the AIMS. An infant's raw score is referred to the distribution of raw scores obtained by the normative sample to discover where he or she ranks in that distribution.

NORMATIVE SAMPLE

A representative birth cohort of all infants born in the province of Alberta, Canada between March 1990 and June 1992 constituted the normative sample for the AIMS. The accessible population included *all* infants—preterm, full-term, and infants with congenital anomalies—who were born in Alberta between March 1990 and June 1992.

Alberta is a western province of Canada with a population of approximately 2.5 million people. All health services in the province are provided through a government-financed national health insurance program. Community health services are delivered on a regional basis in 27 health units distributed geographically within the province.

In order to obtain a sample that was representative of all Albertan infants born over an 18-month period, a two-stage random sampling strategy was employed with health units as the clusters. The final sample was to consist of 2400 infants stratified by age and sex. The average total number of births/year in Alberta is approximately 42,445, distributed among the province's 27 health units as shown in Table 11–1. A map identifying the province's health units is seen in Figure 11–1.

Edmonton and Calgary, as the two largest units, have about one half of the province's births. Therefore, one half of the sample, or 1200 infants, was to be obtained through one randomly selected very large unit—Edmonton. The second 1200 infants were to be drawn from the remaining 25 health units using the following procedure: the health units were grouped into three levels—small, medium, and large—according to their number of births. The strata consisted of 9, 8, and 8 units, respectively. One third of the health units were sampled from each stratum, and random samples of the sizes noted in Table 11–2 were to be drawn from each selected unit. The overall sampling fraction was $1/27$, since the sampling time frame was 18 months.

HEALTH UNITS OF ALBERTA

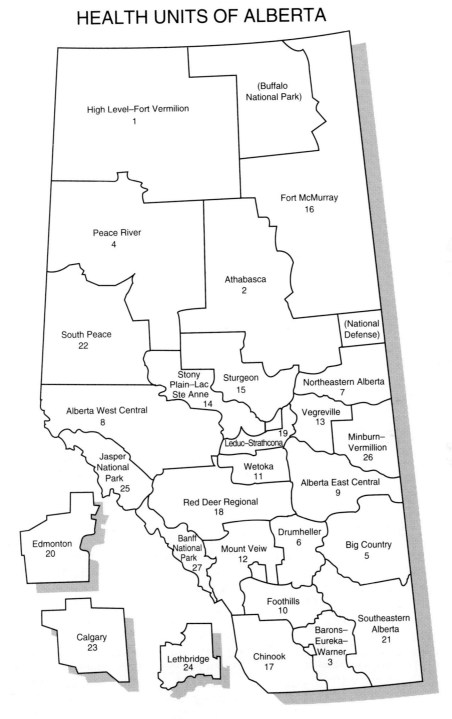

FIGURE 11-1
Health units of Alberta, Canada.

Table 11–1
Health Units—Total Births in 1989

Health Unit (Unit No.)	Births
Edmonton (20)	10,502
Calgary (23)	12,107
East Central (9)	772
Athabasca (2)	672
Banff Park (27)	83
Barons-Eureka-Warner (3)	783
Big Country (5)	185
Chinook (17)	586
Lethbridge (24)	915
Drumheller (6)	528
West Central (8)	758
Foothills (10)	520
Fort-McMurray (16)	708
South Peace (22)	1,086
High Level–Fort Vermilion (1)	450
Jasper Park (25)	65
Leduc-Strathcona (19)	1,550
Southeastern Alberta (21)	1,191
Minburn-Vermilion (26)	376
Mount View (12)	1,066
North Eastern Alberta (7)	964
Peace River (4)	800
Red Deer Regional (18)	2,145
Stony Plain-Lac Ste. Anne (14)	1,131
Sturgeon (15)	1,523
Vegreville (13)	386
Wetoka (11)	593

Before sampling infants within units, the population of infants in each unit was stratified by sex and age. Equal numbers of male and female infants were included within each age category so that separate norms could be developed for these two groups. The literature documents slight sex differences in early motor development, which seems to justify the separate development of norms for boys and girls, but fails to support stratification on other variables such as socioeconomic status (Capute et al., 1985). The stratification

Table 11–2
Sampling Design

	Unit Name (Unit No.)	Estimated Births Over 18 Months	Sample Size	Sampling Fraction
Small Units	Jasper Park (25)	97	10	$\frac{1}{3} \times \frac{1}{9}$
	Big Country (5)	278	31	
	High Level–Fort Vermilion (1)*	675	75	
Medium Units	Athabasca (2)	1008	112	$\frac{1}{3} \times \frac{1}{9}$
	West Central (8)	1125	125	
	Barons-Eureka-Warner (3)	1174	131	
Large Units	North Eastern (7)	1446	161	$\frac{1}{3} \times \frac{1}{9}$
	Southeastern (21)	1787	199	
	Red Deer Regional (18)	3217	356	
Very Large Units	Edmonton (20)	15,753	1200	$\frac{1}{2} \times \frac{1}{13}$
	TOTAL 10 Units		2400	

*This health unit was not able to participate in the project, and Minburn-Vermilion was randomly sampled from the group of small health units.

Table 11–3
Stratification by Age

Age of Infant	No. of Infants
1–2 mo	200
3–4 mo	200
5 mo	200
6 mo	200
7 mo	200
8 mo	200
9 mo	200
10 mo	200
11 mo	150
12 mo	150
13–14 mo	200
15–16 mo	150
17–18 mo	150

by age for the total sample of infants was as indicated in Table 11–3. Because the largest number of items in the AIMS is contained within the 5- to 10-month age period, more infants of these ages were sampled than were infants of the younger or older ages. This procedure minimized the standard error in the final norms tables for these very important age groups.

The total sample size of 2400 was chosen based upon the distribution of age categories shown in Table 11–3. Our original intent was to report normative data for boys and girls separately, as well as to report norms for each age group. We believed that 75 to 100 infants in each of these sampling subgroups was the smallest acceptable number of infants upon which to report "representative" norms.

The Division of Vital Statistics, Department of Health, Province of Alberta provided a random sample of potential participants, according to the following criteria: (1) health unit, (2) sex, and (3) date of birth. Since all births in Alberta are registered with the Division of Vital Statistics within a few weeks of occurrence, this division had the most complete information available concerning the population of Alberta infants. It is standard practice in Alberta for the health units to be given immediate notification by the Division of Vital Statistics of the births occurring in their region.

Because Alberta's confidentiality guidelines preclude the release of infants' names to outside individuals, the lists of infants sampled within each health unit were forwarded from the Division of Vital Statistics to the appropriate health units. An initial telephone contact was made with the parents or guardians by health unit personnel. During this contact, the research was briefly described and a verbal consent was sought to permit a member of the research team to make the contact. This second contact involved a more detailed explanation of the study, a request for written consent from the parent or guardian, and the setting up of an appointment for the assessment. In order to offset those individuals who could not be reached or those individuals who would not consent to participate in the study, the Division of Vital Statistics randomly selected twice the number of infants required for each health unit. Despite this procedure, a final sample of 2202 infants, rather than the proposed 2400, participated in the norm-referencing study.

Each assessment was performed in the health unit by one of six physical therapists experienced in infant motor assessment and trained to an acceptable level of reliability (>.80) in the use of the AIMS.

RAW SCORES AND DERIVED SCORES

Upon careful analyses of the normative data, no gender differences were documented in terms of performance on the AIMS. Table 11–4 presents a summary of the scores according to gender. Because of the lack of quantifiable gender differences, the scores for the entire sample were combined and analyzed according to age only.

The normative data collected on the total AIMS raw scores are presented in Appendix III. For each age month, information is provided in terms of the numbers of infants sampled by sex, as well as the mean raw scores, standard deviations, and standard errors.

In order to ascertain more precisely the infant's exact position with reference to the normative sample, the total AIMS raw score (0 to 58) must be converted into some relative measure or derived score. These derived scores are designed to indicate an individual infant's relative standing in the nor-

Table 11–4
Comparison of Gender AIMS Scores by Age Group

Age Group (mo)	Gender	AIMS Score Mean	AIMS Score SD	t	p Value
0–<1	Boy	4.3	1.5	−0.78	.44
	Girl	4.8	1.2		
1–<2	Boy	7.1	1.9	−0.70	.49
	Girl	7.5	2		
2–<3	Boy	9.9	2.5	0.32	.75
	Girl	9.7	2.4		
3–<4	Boy	12.4	2.9	−0.45	.66
	Girl	12.8	3.7		
4–<5	Boy	18	4.2	0.40	.69
	Girl	17.7	4.1		
5–<6	Boy	23.1	4.6	−0.28	.78
	Girl	23.3	4.9		
6–<7	Boy	28.5	5.4	0.49	.63
	Girl	28.1	5.7		
7–<8	Boy	32.6	6.9	0.66	.51
	Girl	31.9	6.8		
8–<9	Boy	39.2	8.6	−0.96	.34
	Girl	40.3	8.8		
9–<10	Boy	46.4	6.8	1.75	.08
	Girl	44.5	8.1		
10–<11	Boy	49.1	6.1	−0.44	.66
	Girl	49.5	5.7		
11–<12	Boy	51.5	6.4	0.46	.64
	Girl	51	7.8		
12–<13	Boy	54.3	4.4	−0.63	.53
	Girl	54.8	4.6		
13–<14	Boy	55.6	4.6	−0.02	.98
	Girl	55.6	5.5		
14–<15	Boy	57.3	1.3	1.68	.10
	Girl	56.4	2.6		
15–<16	Boy	57.7	0.6	−1.97	.06
	Girl	57.9	0.2		
16–<17	Boy	57.8	0.6	−0.37	.71
	Girl	57.8	0.4		
17–<18	Boy	57.9	0.3	0.81	.42
	Girl	57.8	0.4		
18–<19	Boy	57.6	0.5	−0.72	.48
	Girl	57.8	0.8		

mative sample and thus permit an evaluation of that infant's performance in reference to other age-matched infants.

Derived scores are based on a transformation of the raw score to some other unit of measurement that permits the comparison to the normative sample (Cermak, 1989). There are two ways that raw scores may be converted to derived scores: (1) developmental level attained or (2) relative position within a specified age group (Anastasi, 1988).

In age-equivalent norms, the infant's performance is compared with the performance of infants of many ages, and the resultant age-equivalent score gives an indication at what developmental or age level the infant is performing. For example, a 9-month-old infant who performs as well as the average 11-month-old infant could be described as having a motor performance age equivalence of 11 months.

In within–age group norms, the infant's performance is compared with the performance of the most nearly comparable group of infants in terms of age and then described in terms of the comparable group. For example, the performance of the same 9-month-old infant would be described in terms of other 9-month-old infants.

In the case of the AIMS, the derived scores are reported in terms of within–age group norms through the use of percentile ranks. A percentile rank indicates an individual infant's position relative to the age-matched normative sample. Percentile ranks are expressed in terms of the percentage of infants of a specified age in the normative sample whose scores fall below a given raw score. For example, if a total AIMS raw score of 15 corresponds to the 75th percentile for 3-month-old infants, it means that 75% of 3-month-old infants had raw scores of 15 or less. Similarly, a 3-month-old infant with a score of 15 scored as well as or better than 75% of the 3-month-old infants in the normative sample. With percentiles, the lower the percentile, the less mature the infant's motor development.

The percentile ranks for the total AIMS scores according to age are presented in Appendix II and Appendix IV. Appendix II presents the appropriate percentile ranks associated with every possible total AIMS score by age groupings. These percentile ranks have been determined by calculating the appropriate z-scores (based on the means and standard deviations for the respective age groupings) for each total score. For example, a 6.5-month-old infant who obtains a total AIMS score of 27 is at the 40th percentile for age. Because the percentile ranks listed in Appendix II have been averaged over the entire age month, it is important to recognize that the listed percentiles are less accurate for infants whose age at the time of testing falls at either end of the age month, such as an infant who is 6 months and 2 days or an infant who is 6 months and 28 days old.

Appendix IV provides the total AIMS scores according to age associated with six percentile rankings—that is, the 5th, 10th, 25th, 50th, 75th, and 90th percentiles for each age group of infants. This appendix essentially replicates the developmental graph found in Appendix I that visually depicts the six percentile rankings in graph form. A child's individual total AIMS score may be placed on the developmental graph according to age. Similarly the total AIMS score may be placed between the appropriate percentile rankings as listed in Appendix IV to provide the examiner with an estimate of the percentile ranking of the infant. For example, an infant who is between 4 and 5 months of age and obtains a score of 19 is performing between the 50th and 75th percentiles for age.

APPLICATION OF NORMATIVE DATA—CASE VALIDATION STUDY

The normative data generated for the AIMS have been applied in a case validation study. The basic assumption was made, using the means and standard deviations of the total AIMS scores obtained for each age group, that infants who obtained scores that fell between -1 SD and -2 SD from the mean for a specific age group exhibited "suspicious" motor performance. Similarly, infants who obtained scores that fell below -2 SD from the mean exhibited "abnormal" motor performance (Fig. 11–2).

Although the use of 1 SD and 2 SD as cutoff points to classify infants as suspicious and abnormal is accepted practice with developmental scales, this statistical approach to abnormality, using the properties of normal distribution, may be inappropriate for classifying infants' motor abilities. Motor skills are not categorically abnormal or normal; rather a continuum of severity exists. Predictive abilities might be improved by evaluating a range of cutoff points on a test and choosing the score with the most acceptable combination of sensitivity, specificity, and negative and positive predictive values as the positivity criterion. The age of the infant, the degree of abnormality to be detected, and the consequences of both false-positive and false-negative results should all be considered when assigning cutoff scores. A major predictive validity study is currently being conducted that will be evaluating a variety of cutoff scores for the AIMS. For the purposes of this case validation study, however, 1 SD and 2 SD were employed for classification purposes.

Two groups of infants were assessed using the AIMS: 18 infants with a definitive diagnosis of abnormal motor development and 44 infants who were at risk for motor disorders because of either a gestational age of less than 32 weeks or term asphyxia. Therapists who performed the assessments were unaware of the infants' developmental status and birth history. The results of these assessments were compared with the normative data.

Of the 18 diagnosed abnormal infants, 16 (89%) were considered "abnormal" on the basis of their AIMS scores—that is, they received scores lower than 2 SD below the mean for their respective ages. Two infants obtained

Classification Criteria

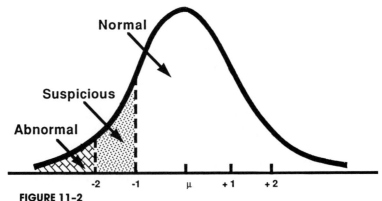

FIGURE 11–2
Use of normative data obtained from the AIMS in a case validation study

Case Validation - Abnormal Babies
(n = 18)

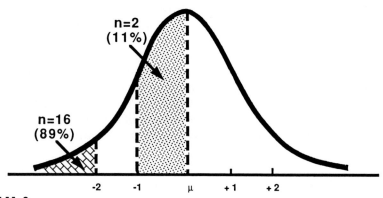

FIGURE 11-3
Graphic representation of data from 18 infants definitively diagnosed as having abnormal motor development.

"normal" scores. The diagnoses of the two abnormal infants who were deemed to be developing normally on the AIMS were Erb's palsy and lipomatous meningomyelocele (Fig. 11–3).

Of the 44 at-risk infants, 10 (23%) were considered to be "suspicious" (between 1 SD and 2 SD below the mean) and 3 (7%) were considered to be "abnormal" (>2 SD below the mean) (Fig. 11–4).

Although the final diagnoses of the at-risk infants are not known at this time, it is clear that these findings concur with the majority of studies to date that suggest that approximately 25 to 30% of at-risk infants will exhibit some form of neuromotor disturbance early in life (Coolman et al., 1985; Piper et al., 1988). It is important to note that an at-risk infant who had been diag-

Case Validation - At-Risk Babies
(n = 44)

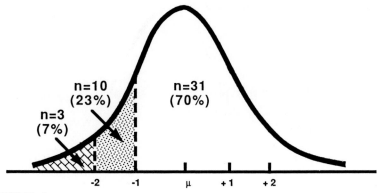

FIGURE 11-4
Graphic representation of data from 44 infants at risk for motor disorders.

nosed very early as having a specific motor disturbance such as spastic quadriplegia, would have been placed in the "abnormal" group of infants rather than our at-risk group, thereby decreasing slightly the number of at-risk infants exhibiting "abnormal" motor development.

These findings suggest that the AIMS is able to accurately discriminate, at the time of testing, those children with abnormal motor development from those who exhibit normal motor development. In addition, the AIMS is able to categorize at-risk infants in the first 18 months of life into three categories: those infants who at the time of testing are exhibiting suspicious patterns of motor development from those who have abnormal or normal patterns of movement. The long-term predictive validity of the AIMS—that is, whether these initial categorizations in the first months of life are predictive of motor outcomes in early childhood, is currently under investigation.

CONCLUSIONS

The AIMS is a norm-referenced test based on age- and sex-stratified normative data collected on a representative sample of 2202 infants born in Alberta. Total AIMS raw scores have been converted to percentile ranks, indicating the infant's position relative to the age-matched normative sample. A case validation study based on the normative data suggests that the AIMS is able to differentiate infants, at the time of testing, into one of three groups: those infants exhibiting abnormal motor development, those infants exhibiting suspicious motor development, and those infants exhibiting normal motor development. The long-term predictive validity of the AIMS is currently under investigation.

References

American Psychological Association: *Standards for Educational and Psychological Tests.* Washington, DC, American Psychological Association, 1983.

Anastasi A: *Psychological Testing,* 6th ed. New York, Macmillan, 1988.

Capute AJ, Shapiro BK, Palmer FB, et al.: Normal gross motor development: the influences of race, sex and socio-economic status. Dev Med Child Neurol 1985; 27:635–643.

Cermak S: Norms and scores. In: Miller LJ (ed): *Developing Norm-Referenced Standardized Tests.* New York, Haworth Press, 1989, pp 91–123.

Coolman, RB, Bennett RC, Sells CJ, et al.: Neuromotor development of graduates of the neonatal intensive care unit: patterns encountered in the first two years of life. J Dev Behav Pediatr 1985; 6:327–333.

Piper MC, Mazer B, Silver KM, et al.: Resolution of neurological symptoms in high-risk infants during the first two years of life. Dev Med Child Neurol 1988; 30:26–35.

APPENDICES

APPENDIX I

PERCENTILE RANKS

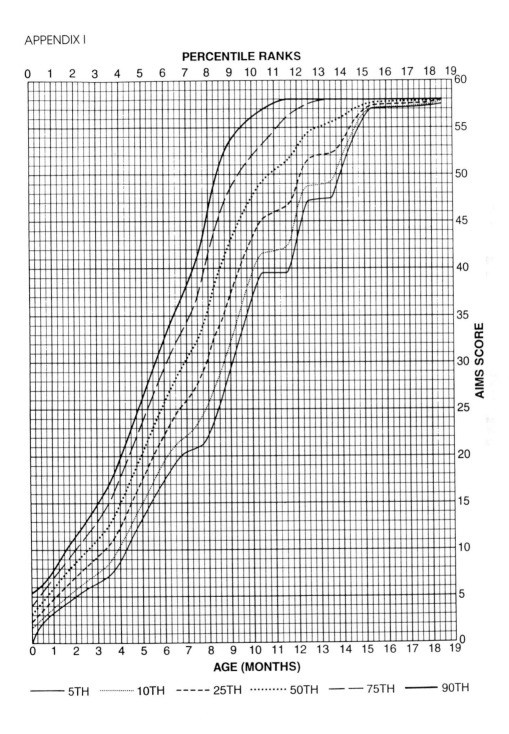

APPENDIX II
Percentile Ranks by Age Grouping

Raw Score							Age in Months									
	≥ 0	1	2	3	4	5	6	7	8	9	10	11	12	13	14
1	1														
2	3														
3	14	1													
4	36	4	1												
5	64	12	2	1											
6	86	25	6	2											
7	97	43	12	5											
8	99	63	23	8	1										
9		80	37	14	2										
10		91	53	22	3										
11		97	69	31	5										
12		99	82	43	8	1									
13			91	55	12	2									
14			96	67	17	3									
15			98	77	24	4									
16			99	85	32	6	1								
17				91	41	10	2	1							
18				95	51	14	3	2							
19				97	60	19	5	3							
20				99	69	25	7	4	1						
21					77	32	9	5	2						
22					84	40	13	7	2						
23					89	48	17	9	3						
24					93	57	22	11	4						
25					96	65	27	15	5						
26					97	72	34	18	6						
27					99	79	41	22	7						
28						84	48	27	9						
29						89	55	32	11	1					
30						92	62	37	13	2					
31						95	69	43	16	3					
32						97	75	48	19	4					
33						98	81	54	22	5					
34						99	85	60	26	6					
35							89	66	29	8	1	1			
36							92	71	33	10	1	2			
37							94	76	38	13	2	2			
38							96	80	42	16	3	3			
39							97	84	46	19	4	4			
40							98	89	51	23	6	6			
41							99	90	56	27	8	8			
42								92	60	32	11	10			
43								94	64	37	14	12			
44								96	69	42	18	15	1	1	
45								97	73	47	23	19	2	2	
46								98	76	52	29	23	3	3	
47								98	80	58	35	27	5	4	
48								99	83	63	41	32	7	6	
49									86	68	48	38	11	9	
50									88	73	54	43	15	13	
51									90	77	61	48	21	18	
52									92	81	67	54	28	24	1
53									94	84	73	60	36	30	2
54									95	87	79	65	45	37	7
55									96	90	83	70	54	45	17
56									97	92	87	75	62	53	32
57									98	94	90	79	70	61	52
58									>98	>95	>93	>83	>77	>68	>71

APPENDIX III
Normative Data

Age (mo)	Male	Female	Total	Mean	SD	SE
0–<1	13	9	22	4.5	1.37	0.19
1–<2	27	29	56	7.3	1.96	0.27
2–<3	60	58	118	9.8	2.42	0.34
3–<4	45	45	90	12.6	3.29	0.46
4–<5	69	53	122	17.9	4.15	0.58
5–<6	80	109	189	23.2	4.75	0.67
6–<7	119	106	225	28.3	5.50	0.77
7–<8	120	102	222	32.3	6.85	0.96
8–<9	109	111	220	39.8	8.69	1.22
9–<10	105	84	189	45.5	7.47	1.05
10–<11	81	74	155	49.3	5.92	0.83
11–<12	77	78	155	51.3	7.11	1
12–<13	53	71	124	54.6	4.52	0.63
13–<14	47	39	86	55.6	5.01	0.7
14–<15	36	25	61	56.9	1.97	0.28
15–<16	19	21	40	57.8	0.45	0.06
16–<17	28	21	49	57.8	0.55	0.08
17–<18	28	21	49	57.9	0.35	0.05
18–<19	14	16	30	57.7	0.64	0.09

APPENDIX IV
Percentile Ranks

Age (mo)	5th	10th	25th	50th	75th	90th
0–<1	2.2	2.7	3.6	4.5	5.4	6.3
1–<2	4.1	4.8	6	7.3	8.6	9.8
2–<3	5.8	6.7	8.2	9.8	11.4	12.9
3–<4	7.2	8.4	10.4	12.6	14.8	16.8
4–<5	11.1	12.6	15.1	17.9	20.7	23.2
5–<6	15.4	17.1	20	23.2	26.4	29.3
6–<7	19.3	21.2	24.6	28.3	32	35.4
7–<8	21	23.5	27.7	32.3	36.9	41.1
8–<9	25.5	28.7	33.9	39.8	45.7	50.9
9–<10	33.2	35.9	40.5	45.5	50.5	55.1
10–<11	39.6	41.7	45.3	49.3	53.3	56.9
11–<12	39.6	42.2	46.5	51.3	56.1	58
12–<13	47.2	48.8	51.6	54.6	57.6	58
13–<14	47.4	49.2	52.2	55.6	58	58
14–<15	53.7	54.4	55.6	56.9	58	58
15–<16	57.1	57.2	57.5	57.8	58	58
16–<17	56.9	57.1	57.4	57.8	58	58
17–<18	57.3	57.5	57.7	57.9	58	58
18–<19	56.6	56.9	57.3	57.7	58	58

Index